The Mediterranean Diet Cookbook:

Tasty Recipes to Kick-Start Your Health Goals.

TABLE OF CONTENTS

THE MEDITERRANEAN DIET COOKBOOK: 1

TASTY RECIPES TO KICK-START YOUR HEALTH GOALS. 1

INTRODUCTION 5

RICE, BEAN, AND GRAIN RECIPES...8

1. LEBANESE RICE AND BROKEN NOODLES WITH CABBAGE......................8
2. LEMON FARRO BOWL WITH AVOCADO 9
3. BARLEY RISOTTO WITH PARMESAN 10
4. GARLIC-ASPARAGUS ISRAELI COUSCOUS 12
5. LENTILS WITH SPINACH AND TOASTED GARLIC 13
6. STEWED OREGANO CHICKPEAS WITH VEGGIES.....................................15
7. HOT CHICKPEAS WITH TURNIPS 16
8. RICH CHICKPEA SALAD...17
9. GOLDEN FALAFEL 18
10. WARM SPICED CRANBERRY BEANS 20
11. RITZY CRANBERRY BEANS 21
12. SICILIAN CANNELLINI BEANS AND ESCAROLE 22
13. CANNELLINI BEAN SALAD 24
14. BEAN BALLS WITH MARINARA 25

SALAD RECIPES...28

15. TOAST WITH SMOKED SALMON, HERBED CREAM CHEESE, AND GREENS 28
16. CRAB MELT WITH AVOCADO AND EGG 29
17. TOMATO CUCUMBER AVOCADO SALAD 30
18. HEALTHY BROCCOLI SALAD 31
19. AVOCADO LIME SHRIMP SALAD 32
20. GRILLED MAHI-MAHI WITH JICAMA SLAW 33
21. MEDITERRANEAN CHICKEN SALAD..34
22. SHRIMP SALAD COCKTAILS 35
23. GARLIC CHIVE CAULIFLOWER MASH 36
24. BEET GREENS WITH PINE NUTS GOAT CHEESE 37
25. KALE SLAW AND STRAWBERRY SALAD + POPPYSEED DRESSING 38

SIDE RECIPES 40

26. CABBAGE AND MUSHROOMS MIX...40
27. LEMON MUSHROOM RICE 40
28. PAPRIKA AND CHIVES POTATOES 41

29. BULGUR, KALE AND CHEESE MIX 42
30. SPICY GREEN BEANS MIX 43
31. BEANS AND RICE 44
32. TOMATO AND MILLET MIX 45
33. QUINOA AND GREENS SALAD 46
34. VEGGIES AND AVOCADO DRESSING 47
35. DILL BEETS SALAD 48
36. BRUSSELS SPROUTS HASH 49
37. ROASTED ASPARAGUS WITH LEMON AND PINE NUTS 50
38. CITRUS SAUTÉED SPINACH 51
39. MASHED CAULIFLOWER 51
40. BROCCOLI WITH GINGER AND GARLIC 52
41. BALSAMIC ROASTED CARROTS 53
42. PARMESAN ZUCCHINI STICKS 54

MAIN RECIPES: VEGETABLE **56**
43. FETA ASPARAGUS SALAD 56
44. SAUTÉED MUSHROOMS 57
45. MUSHROOMS PEAS FARRO 57
46. DELICIOUS CAULIFLOWER RICE 59
47. GRILLED EGGPLANT 60
48. FLAVORFUL ROASTED VEGETABLES 61
49. HEALTHY CARROT SALAD 62
50. BEETROOT & CARROT SALAD 63
51. OLIVE CARROT SALAD 63

MAIN RECIPES: MEAT **65**
52. ROASTED PORK SHOULDER 65
53. HERB ROASTED PORK 65
54. SLOW COOKED BEEF BRISKET 66
55. MEDITERRANEAN BEEF DISH 67
56. BEEF TARTAR 68
57. MEATBALLS AND SAUCE 69
58. ROSEMARY BEEF CHUCK ROAST 70
59. HERB-ROASTED TURKEY BREAST 71
60. CHICKEN SAUSAGE AND PEPPERS 72
61. CHICKEN PICCATA 73
62. CHICKEN WITH ONIONS, POTATOES, FIGS, AND CARROTS 75
63. CHICKEN GYROS WITH TZATZIKI 76
64. GREEK CHICKEN SALAD 77
65. ONE POT GREEK CHICKEN AND LEMON RICE 78
66. BALSAMIC BEEF DISH 80
67. GREEK CHICKEN WITH VEGETABLES AND LEMON VINAIGRETTE 81
68. SIMPLE GRILLED SALMON WITH VEGGIES 82

69.	CAPRESE CHICKEN HASSELBACK STYLE	84
70.	GRILLED CALAMARI WITH LEMON JUICE	85
71.	BACON-WRAPPED CHICKEN	86
72.	BROCCOLI PESTO SPAGHETTI	87

MAIN RECIPES: SEAFOOD 89

73.	CLASSIC ESCABECHE	89
74.	OLIVE OIL-POACHED TUNA	90
75.	FIDEOS WITH SEAFOOD	92
76.	SHRIMP PESTO RICE BOWLS	93
77.	SALMON WITH TOMATOES AND OLIVES	94
78.	BAKED TROUT WITH LEMON	95
79.	SHRIMP AND PEA PAELLA	96
80.	GARLIC SHRIMP WITH ARUGULA PESTO	97
81.	BAKED OYSTERS WITH VEGETABLES	98
82.	CREAMY FISH GRATIN	99
83.	MIXED SEAFOOD DISH	100

SNACK RECIPES 103

84.	WATERMELON FETA & BALSAMIC PIZZA	103
85.	TOMATO AND CHERRY LINGUINE	103
86.	MEDITERRANEAN ZUCCHINI MUSHROOM PASTA	105
87.	LEMON AND GARLIC FETTUCINE	106
88.	ROASTED BROCCOLI WITH PARMESAN	107
89.	SPINACH AND FETA BREAD	108
90.	QUICK ZUCCHINI BOWL	109
91.	HEALTHY BASIL PLATTER	110
92.	CRISPY SWEET POTATO FRIES	112
93.	BAKED EGGS AND ASPARAGUS WITH PARMESAN	112
94.	FLAVORFUL BRAISED KALE	113
95.	BASIL TOMATO SKEWERS	114

DESSERT RECIPES 116

96.	ALMOND COOKIES	116
97.	BAKLAVA AND HONEY	117
98.	BAKED APPLES WITH WALNUTS AND SPICES	118
99.	RED WINE POACHED PEARS	119
100.	VANILLA PUDDING WITH STRAWBERRIES	120
101.	MIXED BERRY FROZEN YOGURT BAR	121

CONCLUSION 123

INTRODUCTION

What is Mediterranean Diet?

Mediterranean Diet is characterized by high consumption of pasta, olive oil, fresh fruits and vegetables. Fish, poultry, legumes, oatmeal, and nuts are also widely eaten, and red meat is consumed in low amounts.

The Benefits of this diet is -

1. Longer life span.
2. Less incidence of depression.
3. Lower incidence of asthma.
4. Lower risk of heart disease.
5. Less arthritis and other degenerative joint disease.
6. Fewer strokes.
7. Better postmenopausal health - lower incidence of bone fractures and hip fractures.
8. Lighter menstrual periods.
9. Lower cholesterol.
10. Higher HDL levels (good cholesterol), which decreases the risk of coronary heart disease.

Mediterranean Diet had become part of the UNESCO World Heritage Site list in 2011 and been recommended by the World Health Organization (WHO) and the United Nations as model for health in the 21st century.

This diet is strongly recommended by doctors because it not only control blood pressure but also stops the problem of heart ailments.

Because of all these reasons, it became very popular in most part of the world.

This diet can reduce your weight. You can stick to it and modify it and enjoy the life with your family. You can also escape from strokes, heart attacks and diabetes.

Are you suffering from fatty liver? Then you also should adopt this diet plan. The meal which is prepared is low in fat content and has less cholesterol.

It improves your immune system and also helps in your growth process.

You can also order this diet online and any place you like. And if you are not convinced then don't hesitate to ask your nutritionist about this diet, she will convince you to take this diet plan.

Before any diet make sure to ask your doctors about it, and if no doctor can do, then you should ask your own experts. It is because in the diet plan, no matter how good it is, you cannot take food if you are allergic to it. And it is a wrong belief that dieting can reduce your weight, most of the time it mutates your body fat in the healthy fat. Because of which you can get hurt if you eat unhealthy food.

Because of a wrong food diet, you can many health problems, so before taking any diet, ask your doctor about it.

Unlike other diets is composed of a varied diet with unprocessed, but seasonal foods, remember what are the most suitable foods and which to avoid, and then you will be able to make your own choice. However, it is also important to pick the best time of the year to do it.

Mediterranean Diet being a being a very varied diet, can become a lifestyle because it is very balanced, unlike other diets that are often linked to the fashion of the moment and tend instead to eliminate only a certain type of food. Precisely for this reason doctors recommend and indicate it as prevention of various diseases such as hypertension, cancer, diabetes, Alzheimer's etc., it is also suitable for athletes because the facts contained within the diet are natural fats such as omega3, then it is very useful because it allows if followed with care and regularity to maintain the ideal weight form, and precisely for this reason it is considered a lifestyle, then it is important to know that this diet is tested and studied by the scientific world since 1940 and therefore we have decades of data available on its benefits.

Overweight and obesity cost the United States $147 billion in medical spending in 2008, with 60% of the spending directly related to obesity.

Mediterranean Diet helps to Lose Weight

Whether you're looking to maintain, lose, or gain weight, there's a Mediterranean diet plan out there for you. The right Mediterranean diet plan can be challenging; one that provides delicious and satisfying meals while still allowing for weight loss and other health benefits. But it doesn't have to be difficult when you use these tips.

A Mediterranean diet does not need to include only foods from the Mediterranean region.

I hope that you will love this book and I wish somebody inspire you and caught your thoughts on health and eating.

RICE, BEAN, AND GRAIN

RECIPES

---

1. Lebanese Rice and Broken Noodles with Cabbage

Preparation time: 5 minutes

Cooking time: 25 minutes

Servings: 6

INGREDIENTS:

- 1 tablespoon extra-virgin olive oil
- 1 cup (about 3 ounces) uncooked vermicelli or thin spaghetti, broken into 1- to 1½-inch pieces
- 3 cups shredded cabbage (about half a 14-ounce package of coleslaw mix or half a small head of cabbage)
- 3 cups low-sodium or no-salt-added vegetable broth
- ½ cup water
- 1 cup instant brown rice
- 2 garlic cloves
- ¼ teaspoon kosher or sea salt
- 1/8 to ¼ teaspoon crushed red pepper
- ½ cup loosely packed, coarsely chopped cilantro

- Fresh lemon slices, for serving (optional)

DIRECTIONS:

1. In a large saucepan over medium-high heat, heat the oil. Add the pasta and cook for 3 minutes to toast, stirring often.

2. Add the cabbage and cook for 4 minutes, stirring often. Add the broth, water, rice, garlic, salt, and crushed red pepper, and bring to a boil over high heat.

3. Stir, cover, and reduce the heat to medium-low. Simmer for 10 minutes. Remove the pan from the heat, but do not lift the lid. Let sit for 5 minutes.

4. Fish out the garlic cloves, mash them with a fork, then stir the garlic back into the rice. Stir in the cilantro. Serve with the lemon slices (if using).

NUTRITION: Calories: 259 Fat: 4g Carbohydrates: 49g Protein: 7g

2. Lemon Farro Bowl with Avocado

Preparation time: 5 minutes

Cooking time: 25 minutes

Servings: 6

INGREDIENTS:

- 1 tablespoon plus 2 teaspoons extra-virgin olive oil, divided
- 1 cup chopped onion (about ½ medium onion)
- 2 garlic cloves, minced (about 1 teaspoon)
- 1 carrot, shredded (about 1 cup)
- 2 cups low-sodium or no-salt-added vegetable broth

- 1 cup (6 ounces) uncooked pearled or 10-minute farro
- 2 avocados, peeled, pitted, and sliced
- 1 small lemon
- ¼ teaspoon kosher or sea salt

DIRECTIONS:

1. In a medium saucepan over medium-high heat, heat 1 tablespoon of oil. Add the onion and cook for 5 minutes, stirring occasionally.

2. Add the garlic and carrot and cook for 1 minute, stirring frequently. Add the broth and farro, and bring to a boil over high heat.

3. Lower the heat to medium-low, cover, and simmer for about 20 minutes or until the farro is plump and slightly chewy (al dente).

4. Pour the farro into a serving bowl, and add the avocado slices. Using a Microplane or citrus zester, zest the peel of the lemon directly into the bowl of farro.

5. Halve the lemon, and squeeze the juice out of both halves using a citrus juicer or your hands. Drizzle the remaining 2 teaspoons of oil over the bowl, and sprinkle with salt. Gently mix all the ingredients and serve.

NUTRITION: Calories: 279 Fat: 14g Carbohydrates: 36g Protein: 7g

3. Barley Risotto with Parmesan

Preparation time: 5 minutes

Cooking time: 25 minutes

Servings: 6

INGREDIENTS:

- 4 cups low-sodium or no-salt-added vegetable broth
- 1 tablespoon extra-virgin olive oil
- 1 cup chopped yellow onion (about ½ medium onion)
- 2 cups uncooked pearl barley
- ½ cup dry white wine
- 1 cup freshly grated Parmesan cheese (about 4 ounces), divided
- ¼ teaspoon kosher or sea salt
- ¼ teaspoon freshly ground black pepper
- Fresh chopped chives and lemon wedges, for serving (optional)

DIRECTIONS:

1. Pour the broth into a medium saucepan and bring to a simmer. In a large stockpot over medium-high heat, heat the oil.
2. Add the onion and cook for 8 minutes, stirring occasionally. Add the barley and cook for 2 minutes, stirring until the barley is toasted.
3. Pour in the wine and cook for about 1 minute, or until most of the liquid evaporates. Add 1 cup of warm broth to the pot and cook, stirring, for about 2 minutes, or until most of the liquid is absorbed.
4. Add the remaining broth 1 cup at a time, cooking until each cup is absorbed (about 2 minutes each time) before adding the next. The last addition of broth will take a bit longer to absorb, about 4 minutes.

5. Remove the pot from the heat, and stir in ½ cup of cheese, and the salt and pepper. Serve with the remaining cheese on the side, along with the chives and lemon wedges (if using).

NUTRITION: Calories: 346 Fat: 7g Carbohydrates: 56g Protein: 14g

4. Garlic-Asparagus Israeli Couscous

Preparation time: 5 minutes

Cooking time: 25 minutes

Servings: 6

INGREDIENTS:

- 1 cup garlic-and-herb goat cheese (about 4 ounces)
- 1½ pounds asparagus spears, ends trimmed and stalks chopped into 1-inch pieces (about 2¾ to 3 cups chopped)
- 1 tablespoon extra-virgin olive oil
- 1 garlic clove, minced (about ½ teaspoon)
- ¼ teaspoon freshly ground black pepper
- 1¾ cups water
- 1 (8-ounce) box uncooked whole-wheat or regular Israeli couscous (about 1⅓ cups)
- ¼ teaspoon kosher or sea salt

DIRECTIONS:

1. Preheat the oven to 425°F. Put the goat cheese on the counter to bring to room temperature.

2. In a large bowl, mix together the asparagus, oil, garlic, and pepper. Spread the asparagus on a large, rimmed baking sheet and roast for 10 minutes, stirring a few times.

3. Remove the pan from the oven, and spoon the asparagus into a large serving bowl. While the asparagus is roasting, in a medium saucepan, bring the water to a boil.

4. Add the couscous and salt. Reduce the heat to medium-low, cover, and cook for 12 minutes, or until the water is absorbed.

5. Pour the hot couscous into the bowl with the asparagus. Add the goat cheese, mix thoroughly until completely melted, and serve.

NUTRITION: Calories: 263 Fat: 9g Carbohydrates: 36g Protein: 11g

5. Lentils with Spinach and Toasted Garlic

Preparation time: 10 minutes

Cooking time: 58 minutes

Servings: 6

INGREDIENTS:

- 2 tablespoons extra-virgin olive oil
- 4 garlic cloves, sliced thin
- Salt and pepper, to taste
- 1 onion, chopped fine
- 1 teaspoon ground coriander
- 1 teaspoon ground cumin
- 2½ cups water

- 1 cup green or brown lentils, picked over and rinsed
- 8 ounces (227 g) curly-leaf spinach, stemmed and chopped coarse
- 1 tablespoon red wine vinegar

DIRECTIONS:

1. Cook oil and garlic in large saucepan over medium-low heat, stirring often, until garlic turns crisp and golden but not brown, about 5 minutes.

2. Using slotted spoon, transfer garlic to paper towel–lined plate and season lightly with salt; set aside.

3. Add onion and ½ teaspoon salt to oil left in saucepan and cook over medium heat until softened and lightly browned, 5 to 7 minutes. Stir in coriander and cumin and cook until fragrant, about 30 seconds.

4. Stir in water and lentils and bring to simmer. Reduce heat to low, cover, and simmer gently, stirring occasionally, until lentils are mostly tender but still intact, 45 to 55 minutes.

5. Stir in spinach, 1 handful at a time. Cook, uncovered, stirring occasionally, until spinach is wilted and lentils are completely tender, about 8 minutes.

6. Stir in vinegar and season with salt and pepper to taste. Transfer to serving dish, sprinkle with toasted garlic, and serve.

NUTRITION: Calories: 160 Carbs: 22g Fat: 5g Protein: 8g

6. Stewed Oregano Chickpeas with Veggies

Preparation time: 15 minutes

Cooking time: 51 minutes

Servings: 6

INGREDIENTS:

- ¼ cup extra-virgin olive oil
- 2 onions, chopped
- 1 green bell pepper, stemmed, seeded, and chopped fine
- Salt and pepper, to taste
- 3 garlic cloves, minced
- 1 tablespoon minced fresh oregano or 1 teaspoon dried
- 2 bay leaves
- 1 pound (454 g) eggplant, cut into 1-inch pieces
- 1 (28-ounce / 794-g) can whole peeled tomatoes, drained with juice reserved, chopped coarse
- 2 (15-ounce / 425-g) cans chickpeas, drained with 1 cup liquid reserved

DIRECTIONS:

1. Adjust oven rack to lower-middle position and heat oven to 400°F (205°C). Heat oil in Dutch oven over medium heat until shimmering.

2. Add onions, bell pepper, ½ teaspoon salt, and ¼ teaspoon pepper and cook until softened, about 5 minutes. Stir in garlic, 1

teaspoon oregano, and bay leaves and cook until fragrant, about 30 seconds.

3. Stir in eggplant, tomatoes and reserved juice, and chickpeas and reserved liquid and bring to boil.

4. Transfer pot to oven and cook, uncovered, until eggplant is very tender, 45 to 60 minutes, stirring twice during cooking.

5. Discard bay leaves. Stir in remaining 2 teaspoons oregano and season with salt and pepper to taste. Serve.

NUTRITION: Calories: 133 Carbs: 20g Fat: 2g Protein: 7g

7. Hot Chickpeas with Turnips

Preparation time: 15 minutes

Cooking time: 31 minutes

Servings: 4-6

INGREDIENTS:

- 2 tablespoons extra-virgin olive oil
- 2 onions, chopped
- 2 red bell peppers, stemmed, seeded, and chopped
- Salt and pepper, to taste
- ¼ cup tomato paste
- 1 jalapeño chili, stemmed, seeded, and minced
- 5 garlic cloves, minced
- ¾ teaspoon ground cumin
- ¼ teaspoon cayenne pepper
- 2 (15-ounce / 425-g) cans chickpeas

- 12 ounces (340 g) turnips, peeled and cut into ½-inch pieces
- ¾ cup water, plus extra as needed
- ¼ cup chopped fresh parsley
- 2 tablespoons lemon juice, plus extra for seasoning

DIRECTIONS:

1. Heat oil in Dutch oven over medium heat until shimmering. Add onions, bell peppers, ½ teaspoon salt, and ¼ teaspoon pepper and cook until softened and lightly browned, 5 to 7 minutes.
2. Stir in tomato paste, jalapeño, garlic, cumin, and cayenne and cook until fragrant, about 30 seconds.
3. Stir in chickpeas and their liquid, turnips, and water. Bring to simmer and cook until turnips are tender and sauce has thickened, 25 to 35 minutes.
4. Stir in parsley and lemon juice. Season with salt, pepper, and extra lemon juice to taste. Adjust consistency with extra hot water as needed. Serve.

NUTRITION: Calories: 62 Carbs: 11g Fat: 2g Protein: 2g

8. Rich Chickpea Salad

Preparation time: 15 minutes

Cooking time: 3 minutes

Servings: 6

INGREDIENTS:

- 2 (15-ounce / 425-g) cans chickpeas, rinsed
- ¼ cup extra-virgin olive oil

- 2 tablespoons lemon juice

- Salt and pepper, to taste

- Pinch cayenne pepper

- 3 carrots, peeled and shredded

- 1 cup baby arugula, chopped coarse

- ½ cup pitted kalamata olives, chopped coarse

DIRECTIONS:

1. Microwave chickpeas in medium bowl until hot, about 2 minutes. Stir in oil, lemon juice, ¾ teaspoon salt, ½ teaspoon pepper, and cayenne and let sit for 30 minutes.

2. Add carrots, arugula, and olives and toss to combine. Season with salt and pepper to taste. Serve.

NUTRITION: Calories: 220 Carbs: 35g Fat: 6g Protein: 9g

9. Golden Falafel

Preparation time: 15 minutes

Cooking time: 6 minutes

Servings: 24

INGREDIENTS:

- Salt and pepper, to taste

- 12 ounces (340 g) dried chickpeas, picked over and rinsed

- 10 scallions, chopped coarse

- 1 cup fresh parsley leaves

- 1 cup fresh cilantro leaves

- 6 garlic cloves, minced

- ½ teaspoon ground cumin
- 1/8 teaspoon ground cinnamon
- 2 cups vegetable oil

DIRECTIONS:

1. Dissolve 3 tablespoons salt in 4 quarts cold water in large container. Add chickpeas and soak at room temperature for at least 8 hours or up to 24 hours. Drain and rinse well.

2. Process chickpeas, scallions, parsley, cilantro, garlic, 1 teaspoon salt, 1 teaspoon pepper, cumin, and cinnamon in food processor until smooth, about 1 minute, scraping down sides of bowl as needed.

3. Pinch off and shape chickpea mixture into 2-tablespoon-size disks, about 1½ inches wide and 1 inch thick, and place on parchment paper–lined baking sheet. (Falafel can be refrigerated for up to 2 hours.)

4. Adjust oven rack to middle position and heat oven to 200°F (93°C). Set wire rack in rimmed baking sheet. Heat oil in 12-inch skillet over medium-high heat to 375°F (190°C).

5. Fry half of falafel until deep golden brown, 2 to 3 minutes per side. Adjust burner, if necessary, to maintain oil temperature of 375°F (190°C).

6. Using slotted spoon, transfer falafel to prepared sheet and keep warm in oven. Return oil to 375°F (190°C) and repeat with remaining falafel. Serve.

NUTRITION: Calories: 81 Carbs: 8g Fat: 3g Protein: 4g

10. Warm Spiced Cranberry Beans

Preparation time: 15 minutes

Cooking time: 1 hour & 30 minutes

Servings: 6-8

INGREDIENTS:

- Salt and pepper, to taste
- 1 pound (454 g) dried cranberry beans, picked over and rinsed
- ¼ cup extra-virgin olive oil
- 1 onion, chopped fine
- 2 carrots, peeled and chopped fine
- 4 garlic cloves, sliced thin
- 1 tablespoon tomato paste
- ½ teaspoon ground cinnamon
- ½ cup dry white wine
- 4 cups chicken or vegetable broth
- 2 tablespoons lemon juice, plus extra for seasoning
- 2 tablespoons minced fresh mint

DIRECTIONS:

1. Dissolve 3 tablespoons salt in 4 quarts cold water in large container. Add beans and soak at room temperature for at least 8 hours or up to 24 hours. Drain and rinse well.

2. Adjust oven rack to lower-middle position and heat oven to 350°F (180°C). Heat oil in Dutch oven over medium heat until shimmering.

3. Add onion and carrots and cook until softened, about 5 minutes. Stir in garlic, tomato paste, cinnamon, and ¼ teaspoon pepper and cook until fragrant, about 1 minute.

4. Stir in wine, scraping up any browned bits. Stir in broth, ½ cup water, and beans and bring to boil. Cover, transfer pot to oven, and cook until beans are tender, about 1½ hours, stirring every 30 minutes.

5. Stir in lemon juice and mint. Season with salt, pepper, and extra lemon juice to taste. Adjust consistency with extra hot water as needed. Serve.

NUTRITION: Calories: 205 Carbs: 24g Fat: 2g Protein: 16g

11. Ritzy Cranberry Beans

Preparation time: 15 minutes

Cooking time: 1 hour & 35 minutes

Servings: 6-8

INGREDIENTS:

- Salt and pepper, to taste
- 1 pound (454 g) dried cranberry beans, picked over and rinsed
- 3 tablespoons extra-virgin olive oil
- ½ fennel bulb, 2 tablespoons fronds chopped, stalks discarded, bulb cored and chopped
- 1 cup plus 2 tablespoons red wine vinegar
- ½ cup sugar
- 1 teaspoon fennel seeds

- 6 ounces (170 g) seedless red grapes, halved
- ½ cup pine nuts, toasted

DIRECTIONS:

1. Dissolve 3 tablespoons salt in 4 quarts cold water in large container. Add beans and soak at room temperature for at least 8 hours or up to 24 hours. Drain and rinse well.

2. Bring beans, 4 quarts water, and 1 teaspoon salt to boil in Dutch oven. Reduce to simmer and cook, stirring occasionally, until beans are tender, 1 to 1½ hours. Drain beans and set aside.

3. Wipe Dutch oven clean with paper towels. Heat oil in now-empty pot over medium heat until shimmering.

4. Add fennel, ¼ teaspoon salt, and ¼ teaspoon pepper and cook until softened, about 5 minutes. Stir in 1 cup vinegar, sugar, and fennel seeds until sugar is dissolved.

5. Bring to simmer and cook until liquid is thickened to syrupy glaze and edges of fennel are beginning to brown, about 10 minutes.

6. Add beans to vinegar-fennel mixture and toss to coat. Transfer to large bowl and let cool to room temperature.

7. Add grapes, pine nuts, fennel fronds, and remaining 2 tablespoons vinegar and toss to combine. Season with salt and pepper to taste and serve.

NUTRITION: Calories: 147 Carbs: 44g Fat: 0g Protein: 15g

12. Sicilian Cannellini Beans and Escarole

Preparation time: 15 minutes

Cooking time: 21 minutes

Servings: 4

INGREDIENTS:

- 1 tablespoon extra-virgin olive oil, plus extra for serving
- 2 onions, chopped fine
- Salt and pepper, to taste
- 4 garlic cloves, minced
- 1/8 teaspoon red pepper flakes
- 1 (1-pound / 454-g) head escarole, trimmed and sliced 1 inch thick
- 1 (15-ounce / 425-g) can cannellini beans, rinsed
- 1 cup chicken or vegetable broth
- 1 cup water
- 2 teaspoons lemon juice

DIRECTIONS:

1. Heat oil in Dutch oven over medium heat until shimmering. Add onions and ½ teaspoon salt and cook until softened and lightly browned, 5 to 7 minutes.
2. Stir in garlic and pepper flakes and cook until fragrant, about 30 seconds. Stir in escarole, beans, broth, and water and bring to simmer.
3. Cook, stirring occasionally, until escarole is wilted, about 5 minutes. Increase heat to high and cook until liquid is nearly evaporated, 10 to 15 minutes.
4. Stir in lemon juice and season with salt and pepper to taste. Drizzle with extra oil and serve.

NUTRITION: Calories: 110 Carbs: 18g Fat: 2g Protein: 5g

13. Cannellini Bean Salad

Preparation time: 15 minutes

Cooking time: 8 minutes

Servings: 6-8

INGREDIENTS:

- ¼ cup extra-virgin olive oil
- 3 garlic cloves, peeled and smashed
- 2 (15-ounce / 425-g) cans cannellini beans, rinsed
- Salt and pepper, to taste
- 2 teaspoons sherry vinegar
- 1 small shallot, minced
- 1 red bell pepper, stemmed, seeded, and cut into ¼-inch pieces
- ¼ cup chopped fresh parsley
- 2 teaspoons chopped fresh chives

DIRECTIONS:

1. Cook 1 tablespoon oil and garlic in medium saucepan over medium heat, stirring often, until garlic turns golden but not brown, about 3 minutes.
2. Add beans, 2 cups water, and 1 teaspoon salt and bring to simmer. Remove from heat, cover, and let sit for 20 minutes.
3. Meanwhile, combine vinegar and shallot in large bowl and let sit for 20 minutes. Drain beans and remove garlic.

4. Add beans, remaining 3 tablespoons oil, bell pepper, parsley, and chives to shallot mixture and gently toss to combine. Season with salt and pepper to taste. Let sit for 20 minutes. Serve.

NUTRITION: Calories: 200 Carbs: 11g Fat: 14g Protein: 10g

14. Bean Balls with Marinara

Preparation time: 15 minutes

Cooking time: 30 minutes

Servings: 2-4

INGREDIENTS:

- Bean Balls:
- 1 tablespoon extra-virgin olive oil
- ½ yellow onion, minced
- 1 teaspoon fennel seeds
- 2 teaspoons dried oregano
- ½ teaspoon crushed red pepper flakes
- 1 teaspoon garlic powder
- 1 (15-ounce / 425-g) can white beans (cannellini or navy), drained and rinsed
- ½ cup whole-grain bread crumbs
- Sea salt and ground black pepper, to taste
- Marinara:
- 1 tablespoon extra-virgin olive oil
- 3 garlic cloves, minced
- Handful basil leaves

- 1 (28-ounce / 794-g) can chopped tomatoes with juice reserved
- Sea salt, to taste

DIRECTIONS:

1. Preheat the oven to 350°F (180°C). Line a baking sheet with parchment paper. Heat the olive oil in a nonstick skillet over medium heat until shimmering.
2. Add the onion and sauté for 5 minutes or until translucent. Sprinkle with fennel seeds, oregano, red pepper flakes, and garlic powder, then cook for 1 minute or until aromatic.
3. Pour the sautéed mixture in a food processor and add the beans and bread crumbs. Sprinkle with salt and ground black pepper, then pulse to combine well and the mixture holds together.
4. Shape the mixture into balls with a 2-ounce (57-g) cookie scoop, then arrange the balls on the baking sheet.
5. Bake in the preheated oven for 30 minutes or until lightly browned. Flip the balls halfway through the cooking time.
6. While baking the bean balls, heat the olive oil in a saucepan over medium-high heat until shimmering. Add the garlic and basil and sauté for 2 minutes or until fragrant.
7. Fold in the tomatoes and juice. Bring to a boil. Reduce the heat to low. Put the lid on and simmer for 15 minutes. Sprinkle with salt.
8. Transfer the bean balls on a large plate and baste with marinara before serving.

NUTRITION: Calories: 351 Fat: 16.4g Protein: 11.5g Carbs: 42.9g

SALAD RECIPES

---

15. Toast with Smoked Salmon, Herbed Cream Cheese, and Greens

Preparation Time: 10 minutes

Cooking Time: 5 minutes

Servings: 2

INGREDIENTS:

- For the herbed cream cheese:
- ¼ cup cream cheese, at room temperature
- 2 tablespoons chopped fresh flat-leaf parsley
- 2 tablespoons chopped fresh chives or sliced scallion
- ½ teaspoon garlic powder
- ¼ teaspoon kosher salt
- For the toast:
- 2 slices bread
- 4 ounces smoked salmon
- Small handful microgreens or sprouts
- 1 tablespoon capers, drained and rinsed
- ¼ small red onion, very thinly sliced

DIRECTIONS:

1. In a medium bowl, combine the cream cheese, parsley, chives, garlic powder, and salt. Using a fork, mix until combined. Chill until ready to use.

2. Toast the bread until golden. Spread the herbed cream cheese over each piece of toast, then top with the smoked salmon. Garnish with the microgreens, capers, and red onion.

NUTRITION: Calories: 194 Fat: 8g Carbs: 2g Protein: 12g

16. Crab Melt with Avocado and Egg

Preparation Time: 15 minutes

Cooking Time: 15 minutes

Servings: 2

INGREDIENTS:

- 2 English muffins, split
- 3 tablespoons butter, divided
- 2 tomatoes, cut into slices
- 1 (4-ounce) can lump crabmeat
- 6 ounces sliced or shredded cheddar cheese
- 4 large eggs
- Kosher salt
- 2 large avocados, halved, pitted, and cut into slices
- Microgreens, for garnish

DIRECTIONS:

1. Preheat the broiler. Toast the English muffin halves. Place the toasted halves, cut-side up, on a baking sheet. Spread 1½

teaspoons of butter evenly over each half, allowing the butter to melt into the crevices.

2. Top each with tomato slices, then divide the crab over each, and finish with the cheese. Broil for about 4 minutes until the cheese melts.

3. Meanwhile, in a medium skillet over medium heat, melt the remaining 1 tablespoon of butter, swirling to coat the bottom of the skillet.

4. Crack the eggs into the skillet, giving ample space for each. Sprinkle with salt. Cook for about 3 minutes.

5. Flip the eggs and cook the other side until the yolks are set to your liking. Place 1 egg on each English muffin half. Top with avocado slices and microgreens.

NUTRITION: Calories: 1221 Fat: 84g Carbs: 2g Protein: 12g

17. <u>Tomato Cucumber Avocado Salad</u>

Preparation Time: 15 minutes

Cooking Time: 0 minutes

Servings: 4

INGREDIENTS:

- 12 oz cherry tomatoes, cut in half
- 5 small cucumbers, chopped
- 3 small avocados, chopped
- ½ tsp ground black pepper
- 2 tbsp olive oil
- 2 tbsp fresh lemon juice

- ¼ cup fresh cilantro, chopped
- 1 tsp sea salt

DIRECTIONS:

1. Add cherry tomatoes, cucumbers, avocados, and cilantro into the large mixing bowl and mix well. Mix together olive oil, lemon juice, black pepper, and salt and pour over salad.
2. Toss well and serve immediately.

NUTRITION: Calories 442 Fat 31 g Carbs 30.3 g Protein 2 g

18. Healthy Broccoli Salad

Preparation Time: 25 minutes

Cooking Time: 0 minutes

Servings: 6

INGREDIENTS:

- 3 cups broccoli, chopped
- 1 tbsp apple cider vinegar
- ½ cup Greek yogurt
- 2 tbsp sunflower seeds
- 3 bacon slices, cooked and chopped
- 1/3 cup onion, sliced
- ¼ tsp stevia

DIRECTIONS:

1. In a mixing bowl, mix together broccoli, onion, and bacon. In a small bowl, mix together yogurt, vinegar, and stevia and pour over broccoli mixture. Stir to combine.

2. Sprinkle sunflower seeds on top of the salad. Store salad in the refrigerator for 30 minutes. Serve and enjoy.

NUTRITION: Calories 90 Fat 9 g Carbs 4 g Protein 2 g

19. Avocado Lime Shrimp Salad

Preparation Time: 15 minutes

Cooking Time: 0 minutes

Servings: 2

INGREDIENTS:

- 14 ounces of jumbo cooked shrimp, peeled and deveined; chopped
- 4 ½ ounces of avocado, diced
- 1 ½ cup of tomato, diced
- ¼ cup of chopped green onion
- ¼ cup of jalapeno with the seeds removed, diced fine
- 1 teaspoon of olive oil
- 2 tablespoons of lime juice
- 1/8 teaspoon of salt
- 1 tablespoon of chopped cilantro

DIRECTIONS:

1. Get a small bowl and combine green onion, olive oil, lime juice, pepper, a pinch of salt. Wait for about 5 minutes for all of them to marinate and mellow the flavor of the onion.

2. Get a large bowl and combined chopped shrimp, tomato, avocado, jalapeno. Combine all of the ingredients, add cilantro, and gently toss. Add pepper and salt as desired.

NUTRITION: Calories: 314 Protein,: 26g Carbs: 15g Fats: 9g

20. Grilled Mahi-Mahi with Jicama Slaw

Preparation Time: 20 minutes

Cooking Time: 10 minutes

Servings: 4

INGREDIENTS:

- 1 teaspoon each for pepper and salt, divided
- 1 tablespoon of lime juice, divided
- 2 tablespoon + 2 teaspoons of extra virgin olive oil
- 4 raw mahi-mahi fillets, which should be about 8 oz. each
- ½ cucumber which should be thinly cut into long strips (it should yield about 1 cup)
- 1 jicama, which should be thinly cut into long strips (it should yield about 3 cups)
- 1 cup of alfalfa sprouts
- 2 cups of coarsely chopped watercress

DIRECTIONS:

1. Combine ½ teaspoon of both pepper and salt, 1 teaspoon of lime juice, and 2 teaspoons of oil in a small bowl. Then brush the mahi-mahi fillets all through with the olive oil mixture.

2. Grill the mahi-mahi on medium-high heat until it becomes done in about 5 minutes, turn it to the other side, and let it be done for about 5 minutes.

3. For the slaw, combine the watercress, cucumber, jicama, and alfalfa sprouts in a bowl. Now combine ½ teaspoon of both pepper and salt, 2 teaspoons of lime juice, and 2 tablespoons of extra virgin oil in a small bowl. Drizzle it over slaw and toss together to combine.

NUTRITION: Calories: 320 Protein: 44g Carbohydrate: 10g Fat: 11 g

21. **Mediterranean Chicken Salad**

Preparation Time: 5 minutes

Cooking Time: 25 minutes

Servings: 4

INGREDIENTS:

- For Chicken:
- 1 ¾ lb. boneless, skinless chicken breast
- ¼ teaspoon each of pepper and salt (or as desired)
- 1 ½ tablespoon of butter, melted
- For Mediterranean salad:
- 1 cup of sliced cucumber
- 6 cups of romaine lettuce, that is torn or roughly chopped
- 10 pitted Kalamata olives
- 1 pint of cherry tomatoes
- 1/3 cup of reduced-fat feta cheese

- ¼ teaspoon each of pepper and salt (or lesser)
- 1 small lemon juice (it should be about 2 tablespoons)

DIRECTIONS:

1. Preheat your oven or grill to about 350F. Season the chicken with salt, butter, and black pepper. Roast or grill chicken until it reaches an internal temperature of 1650F in about 25 minutes.

2. Once your chicken breasts are cooked, remove and keep aside to rest for about 5 minutes before you slice it.

3. Combine all the salad ingredients you have and toss everything together very well. Serve the chicken with Mediterranean salad.

NUTRITION: Calories: 340 Protein: 45g Carbohydrate: 9g Fat: 4 g

22. Shrimp Salad Cocktails

Preparation Time: 35 minutes

Cooking Time: 35 minutes

Servings: 8

INGREDIENTS:

- 2 cups mayonnaise
- 6 plum tomatoes, seeded and finely chopped
- 1/4 cup ketchup
- 1/4 cup lemon juice
- 2 cups seedless red and green grapes, halved
- 1 tablespoon. Worcestershire sauce
- 2 lbs. peeled and deveined cooked large shrimp
- 2 celery ribs, finely chopped

- 3 tablespoons. minced fresh tarragon or 3 teaspoon dried tarragon
- salt and 1/4 teaspoon pepper
- shredded 2 of cups romaine
- papaya or 1/2 cup peeled chopped mango
- parsley or minced chives

DIRECTIONS:

1. Combine Worcestershire sauce, lemon juice, ketchup and mayonnaise together in a small bowl. Combine pepper, salt, tarragon, celery and shrimp together in a large bowl.
2. Put in 1 cup of dressing toss well to coat. Scoop 1 tablespoon. of the dressing into 8 cocktail glasses.
3. Layer each glass with 1/4 cup of lettuce, followed by 1/2 cup of the shrimp mixture, 1/4 cup of grapes, 1/3 cup of tomatoes and finally 1 tablespoon. of mango.
4. Spread the remaining dressing over top; sprinkle chives on top. Serve immediately.

NUTRITION: Calories: 580 Carbohydrate: 16 g Fat: 46 g Protein: 24 g

23. Garlic Chive Cauliflower Mash

Preparation Time: 20 minutes

Cooking Time: 18 minutes

Servings: 5

INGREDIENTS:

- 4 cups cauliflower

- 1/3 cup vegetarian mayonnaise
- 1 garlic clove
- 1/2 teaspoon. kosher salt
- 1 tablespoon. water
- 1/8 teaspoon. pepper
- 1/4 teaspoon. lemon juice
- 1/2 teaspoon lemon zest
- 1 tablespoon Chives, minced

DIRECTIONS:

1. In a bowl that is save to microwave, add the cauliflower, mayo, garlic, water, and salt/pepper and mix until the cauliflower is well coated. Cook on high for 15-18 minutes, until the cauliflower is almost mushy.

2. Blend the mixture in a strong blender until completely smooth, adding a little more water if the mixture is too chunky. Season with the remaining ingredients and serve.

NUTRITION: Calories: 178 Carbohydrate: 14 g Fat: 18 g Protein: 2 g

24. Beet Greens with Pine Nuts Goat Cheese

Preparation Time: 25 minutes

Cooking Time: 15 minutes

Servings: 3

INGREDIENTS:

- 4 cups beet tops, washed and chopped roughly

- 1 teaspoon. EVOO
- 1 tablespoon. no sugar added balsamic vinegar
- 2 oz. crumbled dry goat cheese
- 2 tablespoons. Toasted pine nuts

DIRECTIONS:

1. Warm the oil in a pan, then cook the beet greens on medium high heat until they release their moisture. Let it cook until almost tender.

2. Flavor with salt and pepper and remove from heat. Toss the greens in a mixture of balsamic vinegar and olive oil, then top with the nuts and cheese. Serve warm.

NUTRITION: Calories: 215 Carbohydrate: 4 g Fat: 18 g Protein: 10 g

25. Kale Slaw and Strawberry Salad + Poppyseed Dressing

Preparation Time: 10 minutes

Cooking Time: 20 minutes

Servings: 2

INGREDIENTS:

- Chicken breast; 8 ounces; sliced and baked
- Kale; 1 cup; chopped
- Slaw mix; 1 cup (cabbage, broccoli slaw, carrots mixed)
- Slivered almonds; 1/4 cup
- Strawberries; 1 cup; sliced
- For the dressing:

- Light mayonnaise; 1 tablespoon
- Dijon mustard
- Olive oil; 1 tablespoon
- Apple cider vinegar; 1 tablespoon
- Lemon juice; 1/2 teaspoon
- 1 tablespoon of honey
- Onion powder; 1/4 teaspoon
- Garlic powder; 1/4 teaspoon
- Poppyseeds

DIRECTIONS:

1. Whisk the dressing ingredients together until well mixed, then leave to cool in the fridge. Slice the chicken breasts.
2. Divide 2 bowls of spinach, slaw, and strawberries. Cover with a sliced breast of chicken (4 oz. each), then scatter with almonds. Divide the dressing between the two bowls and drizzle.

NUTRITION: Calories: 150 Carbs: 17g Fat: 1g Protein: 7g

SIDE RECIPES

26. Cabbage and Mushrooms Mix

Preparation time: 10 minutes

Cooking time: 15 minutes

Servings: 2

INGREDIENTS:

- 1 yellow onion, sliced
- 2 tablespoons olive oil
- 1 tablespoon balsamic vinegar
- ½ pound white mushrooms, sliced
- 1 green cabbage head, shredded
- 4 spring onions, chopped
- Salt and black pepper to the taste

DIRECTIONS:

1. Heat up a pan with the oil over medium heat, add the yellow onion and the spring onions and cook for 5 minutes.
2. Add the rest of the ingredients, cook everything for 10 minutes, divide between plates and serve.

NUTRITION: Calories 199 Fat 4.5g Carbs 5.6g Protein 2.2g

27. Lemon Mushroom Rice

Preparation time: 10 minutes

Cooking time: 30 minutes

Servings: 4

INGREDIENTS:

- 2 cups chicken stock
- 1 yellow onion, chopped
- ½ pound white mushrooms, sliced
- 2 garlic cloves, minced
- 8 ounces wild rice
- Juice and zest of 1 lemon
- 1 tablespoon chives, chopped
- 6 tablespoons goat cheese, crumbled
- Salt and black pepper to the taste

DIRECTIONS:

1. Heat up a pot with the stock over medium heat, add the rice, onion and the rest of the ingredients except the chives and the cheese, bring to a simmer and cook for 25 minutes.
2. Add the remaining ingredients, cook everything for 5 minutes, divide between plates and serve as a side dish.

NUTRITION: Calories 222 Fat 5.5g Carbs 12.3g Protein 5.6g

28. Paprika and Chives Potatoes

Preparation time: 10 minutes

Cooking time: 1 hour and 8 minutes

Servings: 4

INGREDIENTS:

- 4 potatoes, scrubbed and pricked with a fork
- 1 tablespoon olive oil
- 1 celery stalk, chopped
- 2 tomatoes, chopped
- 1 teaspoon sweet paprika
- Salt and black pepper to the taste
- 2 tablespoons chives, chopped

DIRECTIONS:

1. Arrange the potatoes on a baking sheet lined with parchment paper, introduce in the oven and bake at 350 degrees F for 1 hour.
2. Cool the potatoes down, peel and cut them into larger cubes. Heat up a pan with the oil over medium heat, add the celery and the tomatoes and sauté for 2 minutes.
3. Add the potatoes and the rest of the ingredients, toss, cook everything for 6 minutes, divide the mix between plates and serve as a side dish.

NUTRITION: Calories 233 Fat 8.7g Carbs 14.4g Protein 6.4g

29. Bulgur, Kale and Cheese Mix

Preparation time: 10 minutes

Cooking time: 10 minutes

Servings: 6

INGREDIENTS:

- 4 ounces bulgur

- 4 ounces kale, chopped
- 1 tablespoon mint, chopped
- 3 spring onions, chopped
- 1 cucumber, chopped
- A pinch of allspice, ground
- 2 tablespoons olive oil
- Zest and juice of ½ lemon
- 4 ounces feta cheese, crumbled

DIRECTIONS:

1. Put bulgur in a bowl, cover with hot water, aside for 10 minutes and fluff with a fork. Heat up a pan with the oil over medium heat, add the onions and the allspice and cook for 3 minutes.
2. Add the bulgur and the rest of the ingredients, cook everything for 5-6 minutes more, divide between plates and serve.

NUTRITION: Calories 200 Fat 6.7g Carbs 15.4g Protein 4.5g

30. Spicy Green Beans Mix

Preparation time: 5 minutes

Cooking time: 15 minutes

Servings: 4

INGREDIENTS:

- 4 teaspoons olive oil
- 1 garlic clove, minced
- ½ teaspoon hot paprika
- ¾ cup veggie stock

- 1 yellow onion, sliced
- 1-pound green beans, trimmed and halved
- ½ cup goat cheese, shredded
- 2 teaspoon balsamic vinegar

DIRECTIONS:

1. Heat up a pan with the oil over medium heat, add the garlic, stir and cook for 1 minute.
2. Add the green beans and the rest of the ingredients, toss, cook everything for 15 minutes more, divide between plates and serve as a side dish.

NUTRITION: Calories 188 Fat 4g Carbs 12.4g Protein 4.4g

31. Beans and Rice

Preparation time: 10 minutes

Cooking time: 55 minutes

Servings: 6

INGREDIENTS:

- 1 tablespoon olive oil
- 1 yellow onion, chopped
- 2 celery stalks, chopped
- 2 garlic cloves, minced
- 2 cups brown rice
- 1 and ½ cup canned black beans, rinsed and drained
- 4 cups water
- Salt and black pepper to the taste

DIRECTIONS:

1. Heat up a pan with the oil over medium heat, add the celery, garlic and the onion, stir and cook for 10 minutes.

2. Add the rest of the ingredients, stir, bring to a simmer and cook over medium heat for 45 minutes. Divide between plates and serve.

NUTRITION: Calories 224 Fat 8.4g Carbs 15.3g Protein 6.2g

32. Tomato and Millet Mix

Preparation time: 10 minutes

Cooking time: 20 minutes

Servings: 6

INGREDIENTS:

- 3 tablespoons olive oil
- 1 cup millet
- 2 spring onions, chopped
- 2 tomatoes, chopped
- ½ cup cilantro, chopped
- 1 teaspoon chili paste
- 6 cups cold water
- ½ cup lemon juice
- Salt and black pepper to the taste

DIRECTIONS:

1. Heat up a pan with the oil over medium heat, add the millet, stir and cook for 4 minutes. Add the water, salt and pepper, stir, bring to a simmer over medium heat cook for 15 minutes.
2. Add the rest of the ingredients, toss, divide the mix between plates and serve as a side dish.

NUTRITION: Calories 222 Fat 10.2g Carbs 14.5g Protein 2.4g

33. Quinoa and Greens Salad

Preparation time: 10 minutes

Cooking time: 0 minutes

Servings: 4

INGREDIENTS:

- 1 cup quinoa, cooked
- 1 medium bunch collard greens, chopped
- 4 tablespoons walnuts, chopped
- 2 tablespoons balsamic vinegar
- 4 tablespoons tahini paste
- 4 tablespoons cold water
- A pinch of salt and black pepper
- 1 tablespoon olive oil

DIRECTIONS:

1. In a bowl, mix the tahini with the water and vinegar and whisk.
2. In a bowl, mix the quinoa with the rest of the ingredients and the tahini dressing, toss, divide the mix between plates and serve as a side dish.

NUTRITION: Calories 175 Fat 3g Carbs 5g Protein 3g

34. Veggies and Avocado Dressing

Preparation time: 10 minutes

Cooking time: 0 minutes

Servings: 4

INGREDIENTS:

- 3 tablespoons pepitas, roasted
- 3 cups water
- 2 tablespoons cilantro, chopped
- 4 tablespoons parsley, chopped
- 1 and ½ cups corn
- 1 cup radish, sliced
- 2 avocados, peeled, pitted and chopped
- 2 mangos, peeled and chopped
- 3 tablespoons olive oil
- 4 tablespoons Greek yogurt
- 1 teaspoon balsamic vinegar
- 2 tablespoons lime juice
- Salt and black pepper to the taste

DIRECTIONS:

1. In your blender, mix the olive oil with avocados, salt, pepper, lime juice, the yogurt and the vinegar and pulse.

2. In a bowl, mix the pepitas with the cilantro, parsley and the rest of the ingredients, and toss. Add the avocado dressing, toss, divide the mix between plates and serve as a side dish.

NUTRITION: Calories 403 Fat 30.5g Carbs 23.5g Protein 3.5g

35. Dill Beets Salad

Preparation time: 10 minutes

Cooking time: 0 minutes

Servings: 6

INGREDIENTS:

- 2 pounds beets, cooked, peeled and cubed
- 2 tablespoons olive oil
- 1 tablespoon lemon juice
- 2 tablespoons balsamic vinegar
- 1 cup feta cheese, crumbled
- 3 small garlic cloves, minced
- 4 green onions, chopped
- 5 tablespoons parsley, chopped
- Salt and black pepper to the taste

DIRECTIONS:

1. In a bowl, mix the beets with the oil, lemon juice and the rest of the ingredients, toss and serve as a side dish.

NUTRITION: Calories 268 Fat 15.5g Carbs 25.7g Protein 9.6g

36. Brussels Sprouts Hash

Preparation time: 10 minutes

Cooking time: 20 minutes

Servings: 4

INGREDIENTS:

- 3 tablespoons extra-virgin olive oil
- 1 onion, finely chopped
- 1 pound Brussels sprouts, bottoms trimmed off, shredded (see tip)
- ½ teaspoon caraway seeds
- ½ teaspoon sea salt
- 1/8 teaspoon freshly ground black pepper
- ¼ cup red wine vinegar
- 1 tablespoon Dijon mustard
- 1 tablespoon honey
- 3 garlic cloves, minced

DIRECTIONS:

2. In a large skillet over medium-high heat, heat the olive oil until it shimmers. Add the onion, Brussels sprouts, caraway seeds, sea salt, and pepper.

3. Cook for 7 to 10 minutes, stirring occasionally, until the Brussels sprouts begin to brown. While the Brussels sprouts cook, whisk the vinegar, mustard, and honey in a small bowl and set aside.

4. Add the garlic to the skillet and cook for 30 seconds, stirring constantly. Add the vinegar mixture to the skillet. Cook for about 5 minutes, stirring, until the liquid reduces by half.

NUTRITION: Calories: 176 Protein: 11g Carbohydrates: 19g Fat: 11g

37. Roasted Asparagus with Lemon and Pine Nuts

Preparation time: 5 minutes

Cooking time: 20 minutes

Servings: 4

INGREDIENTS:

- 1 pound asparagus, trimmed
- 2 tablespoons extra-virgin olive oil
- Juice of 1 lemon
- Zest of 1 lemon
- ¼ cup pine nuts
- ½ teaspoon sea salt
- 1/8 teaspoon freshly ground black pepper

DIRECTIONS:

1. Preheat the oven to 425°F. In a large bowl, toss the asparagus with the olive oil, lemon juice and zest, pine nuts, sea salt, and pepper.
2. Spread in a roasting pan in an even layer. Roast for about 20 minutes until the asparagus is browned.

NUTRITION: Calories: 144 Protein: 4g Carbohydrates: 6g Fat: 13g

38. Citrus Sautéed Spinach

Preparation time: 5 minutes

Cooking time: 5 minutes

Servings: 4

INGREDIENTS:

1. 2 tablespoons extra-virgin olive oil
2. 4 cups fresh baby spinach
3. 1 teaspoon orange zest
4. ¼ cup freshly squeezed orange juice
5. ½ teaspoon sea salt
6. 1/8 teaspoon freshly ground black pepper

DIRECTIONS:

1. In a large skillet over medium-high heat, heat the olive oil until it shimmers. Add the spinach and orange zest. Cook for about 3 minutes, stirring occasionally, until the spinach wilts.
2. Stir in the orange juice, sea salt, and pepper. Cook for 2 minutes more, stirring occasionally. Serve hot.

NUTRITION: Calories: 74 Protein: 7g Carbohydrates: 3g Fat: 7g

39. Mashed Cauliflower

Preparation time: 10 minutes

Cooking time: 15 minutes

Servings: 4

INGREDIENTS:

- 4 cups cauliflower florets

- ¼ cup skim milk
- ¼ cup (2 ounces) grated Parmesan cheese
- 2 tablespoons butter
- 2 tablespoons extra-virgin olive oil
- ½ teaspoon sea salt
- 1/8 teaspoon freshly ground black pepper

DIRECTIONS:

1. In a large pot over medium-high, cover the cauliflower with water and bring it to a boil. Reduce the heat to medium-low, cover, and simmer for about 10 minutes until the cauliflower is soft.

2. Drain the cauliflower and return it to the pot. Add the milk, cheese, butter, olive oil, sea salt, and pepper. Using a potato masher, mash until smooth.

NUTRITION: Calories: 187 Protein: 7g Carbohydrates: 7g Fat: 16g

40. Broccoli with Ginger and Garlic

Preparation time: 10 minutes

Cooking time: 11 minutes

Servings: 4

INGREDIENTS:

- 2 tablespoons extra-virgin olive oil
- 2 cups broccoli florets
- 1 tablespoon grated fresh ginger
- ½ teaspoon sea salt

- 1/8 teaspoon freshly ground black pepper
- 3 garlic cloves, minced

DIRECTIONS:

1. In a large skillet over medium-high heat, heat the olive oil until it shimmers. Add the broccoli, ginger, sea salt, and pepper.

2. Cook for about 10 minutes, stirring occasionally, until the broccoli is soft and starts to brown. Add the garlic and cook for 30 seconds, stirring constantly. Remove from the heat and serve.

NUTRITION: Calories: 80 Protein: 1g Carbohydrates: 4g Fat: 0g

41. Balsamic Roasted Carrots

Preparation time: 10 minutes

Cooking time: 30 minutes

Servings: 4

INGREDIENTS:

- 1½ pounds carrots, quartered lengthwise
- 2 tablespoons extra-virgin olive oil
- ¼ teaspoon sea salt
- 1/8 teaspoon freshly ground black pepper
- 3 tablespoons balsamic vinegar

DIRECTIONS:

1. Preheat the oven to 425°F. In a large bowl, toss the carrots with the olive oil, sea salt, and pepper. Place in a single layer in a roasting pan or on a rimmed baking sheet.

2. Roast for 20 to 30 minutes until the carrots are caramelized. Toss with the vinegar and serve.

NUTRITION: Calories: 132 Protein: 1g Carbohydrates: 17g Fat: 7g

42. **Parmesan Zucchini Sticks**

Preparation time: 10 minutes

Cooking time: 20 minutes

Servings: 4

INGREDIENTs:

- 4 zucchinis, quartered lengthwise
- 2 tablespoons extra-virgin olive oil
- ½ cup (4 ounces) grated Parmesan cheese
- 1 tablespoon Italian seasoning
- ½ teaspoon sea salt
- ¼ teaspoon garlic powder
- 1/8 teaspoon freshly ground black pepper

DIRECTIONS:

1. Preheat the oven to 350°F. In a large bowl, toss the zucchini with the olive oil. In a small bowl, whisk the cheese, Italian seasoning, sea salt, garlic powder, and pepper. Toss with the zucchini.

2. Place the zucchini in a single layer on a rimmed baking sheet. Bake for 15 to 20 minutes until the zucchini is soft.

3. Set the oven to broil, and broil for 1 to 2 minutes until the cheese-herb coating crisps, watching carefully so it doesn't burn.

NUTRITION: Calories: 194 Protein: 12g Carbohydrates: 8g Fat: 14g

MAIN RECIPES:

VEGETABLE

---

43. Feta Asparagus Salad

Preparation time: 10 minutes

Cooking time: 10 minutes

Servings: 4

INGREDIENTS:

- 2 lb. asparagus, ends trimmed
- ¾ cup feta cheese, crumbled
- 1 tbsp lemon juice
- 1 lemon zest
- 3 tbsp olive oil
- ¼ tsp pepper
- ¼ tsp salt

DIRECTIONS:

1. Preheat the grill to high. Arrange asparagus on a foil-lined baking sheet. Drizzle with 2 tablespoons of oil and season with pepper and salt.
2. Place asparagus on the grill and cook for 3-4 minutes. Chop grilled asparagus and transfer to the mixing bowl.

3. Add remaining ingredients to the mixing bowl and toss well. Serve and enjoy.

NUTRITION: Calories: 211 Fat: 16.8g Protein: 9g Carbs: 10.1g

44. Sautéed Mushrooms

Preparation time: 10 minutes

Cooking time: 10 minutes

Servings: 2

INGREDIENTS:

- 10 oz mushrooms, sliced
- 1 tbsp garlic, minced
- ¼ tsp dried thyme
- ¼ cup olive oil
- Pepper
- Salt

DIRECTIONS:

1. Heat 2 tablespoons of oil in a pan over medium heat. Add mushrooms, garlic, thyme, pepper, and salt and sauté mushrooms until tender. Drizzle remaining oil and serve.

NUTRITION: Calories: 253 Fat: 25.6g Protein: 4.7g Carbs: 6.2g

45. Mushrooms Peas Farro

Preparation time: 10 minutes

Cooking time: 30 minutes

Servings: 4

INGREDIENTS:

- 1 cup Italian pearled farro
- ¼ cup fresh mint leaves, chopped
- ½ cup parmesan cheese, grated
- 2 ¼ cup vegetable broth
- 2 thyme sprigs
- 1 tsp paprika
- 1 tsp garlic, minced
- 1 cup frozen peas
- 8 oz mushrooms, sliced
- ¼ cup green onions, chopped
- 2 tbsp olive oil
- Pepper
- Salt

DIRECTIONS:

1. Heat oil in a saucepan over medium-high heat. Add peas, mushrooms, and green onions and sauté for 3-4 minutes. Add garlic sauté for 30 seconds.
2. Add faro, thyme, paprika, pepper, and salt and sauté for 4-5 minutes. Add broth and stir everything well. Bring to boil.
3. Turn heat to medium-low. Cover and cook for 20 minutes or until all liquid is absorbed. Remove saucepan from heat.
4. Add mint leaves and parmesan cheese and stir well. Serve and enjoy.

NUTRITION: Calories: 422 Fat: 14.7g Protein: 26g Carbs: 44.6g

46. Delicious Cauliflower Rice

Preparation time: 10 minutes

Cooking time: 15 minutes

Servings: 4

INGREDIENTS:

- 10 oz cauliflower rice
- 3 tbsp sun-dried tomatoes, minced
- 2 cups spinach, chopped
- 1/3 cup vegetable broth
- 2 tomatoes, diced
- 1 small zucchini, sliced
- 1 garlic clove, minced
- 1 cup mushrooms, sliced
- ½ small onion, diced
- 2 tbsp olive oil
- Pepper
- Salt

DIRECTIONS:

1. Heat oil in a pan over medium heat. Add mushrooms and onion and sauté for 5 minutes. Add garlic and sauté for a minute.
2. Add cauliflower rice, tomato, zucchini, and broth and stir well. Cover and cook for 5 minutes or until all liquid evaporates.
3. Add sun-dried tomatoes and spinach and cook for 3-4 minutes. Season with pepper and salt. Serve and enjoy.

NUTRITION: Calories: 107 Fat: 7.5g Protein: 3.8g Carbs: 9.1g

47. Grilled Eggplant

Preparation time: 10 minutes

Cooking time: 10 minutes

Servings: 4

INGREDIENTS:

- 2 large eggplants, sliced ¼-inch thick
- ½ lemon juice
- 2 tbsp fresh parsley, chopped
- ¼ cup feta cheese, crumbled
- ¼ tsp chili flakes
- 1 tsp dried oregano
- ½ cup olive oil
- Pepper
- Salt

DIRECTIONS:

1. Heat grill pan over medium-high heat. In a small bowl, mix together oil, chili flakes, and oregano. Brush eggplants with oil mixture and season with pepper and salt.

2. Place eggplant slices in a grill pan and cook for 3 minutes per side. Transfer grill eggplant slices on serving dish. Drizzle with lemon juice. Top with feta cheese and parsley. Serve and enjoy.

NUTRITION: Calories: 313 Fat: 27.8g Protein: 4.2g Carbs: 17g

48. Flavorful Roasted Vegetables

Preparation time: 10 minutes

Cooking time: 30 minutes

Servings: 6

INGREDIENTS:

- 1 eggplant, sliced
- 5 fresh basil leaves, sliced
- 2 tsp Italian seasoning
- 2 tbsp olive oil
- 1 onion, sliced
- 1 bell pepper, cut into strips
- 2 zucchinis, sliced
- 2 tomatoes, quartered
- Pepper
- Salt

DIRECTIONS:

1. Preheat the oven to 400 F/ 200 C. Line baking tray with parchment paper. Add all ingredients except basil leaves into the mixing bowl and toss well.

2. Transfer veggie mixture on a prepared baking tray and roast in preheated oven for 30 minutes. Garnish with basil leaves and serve.

NUTRITION: Calories: 95 Fat: 5.5g Protein: 2.3g Carbs: 11.7g

49. Healthy Carrot Salad

Preparation time: 10 minutes

Cooking time: 5 minutes

Servings: 4

INGREDIENTS:

- 1 lb. carrots, peeled and grated
- 1 tsp garlic, minced
- 1 tbsp lemon zest
- ¼ cup fresh lemon juice
- 2 tbsp olive oil
- ¼ tsp cinnamon
- 1 tsp cumin
- 1 tsp sweet paprika
- ¼ cup fresh cilantro, chopped
- ¼ cup fresh parsley, chopped
- ½ cup fresh mint, chopped
- Pepper
- Salt

DIRECTIONS:

1. Add all ingredients into the mixing bowl and mix until well combined. Serve and enjoy.

NUTRITION: Calories: 123 Fat: 7.4g Protein: 1.8g Carbs: 13.9g

50. Beetroot & Carrot Salad

Preparation time: 10 minutes

Cooking time: 5 minutes

Servings: 4

INGREDIENTS:

- 12 oz beetroot, peeled, trimmed, & grated
- 12 oz carrots, peeled, trimmed, & grated
- ¼ cup fresh parsley, chopped
- 1 tbsp red wine vinegar
- 2 tbsp olive oil
- 2 tsp cumin seeds
- 2 shallots, chopped

DIRECTIONS:

1. Heat oil in a pan over medium heat. Once the oil is hot then add cumin seeds and cook for 30 seconds.
2. Remove pan from heat. Add remaining ingredients to the pan and mix well. Serve and enjoy.

NUTRITION: Calories: 138 Fat: 7.4g Protein: 2.4g Carbs: 17.6g

51. Olive Carrot Salad

Preparation time: 10 minutes

Cooking time: 5 minutes

Servings: 4

INGREDIENTS:

- 1 lb. carrots, peeled, sliced 1/8-inch thick

- ½ cup feta cheese, crumbled
- ½ cup fresh Italian parsley, chopped
- ½ cup olives, pitted
- ¼ tsp dried oregano
- ½ tsp dried basil
- ¼ cup olive oil
- ¼ cup fresh lemon juice
- 1 tsp garlic, minced

DIRECTIONS:

1. Add all ingredients into the mixing bowl and toss well. Serve and enjoy.

NUTRITION: Calories: 231 Fat: 18.6g Protein: 4.1g Carbs: 14.1g

MAIN RECIPES: MEAT

52. Roasted Pork Shoulder

Preparation time: 30 minutes

Cooking time: 4 hours

Servings: 6

INGREDIENTS:

- 3 tablespoons garlic, minced
- 3 tablespoons olive oil
- 4 pounds pork shoulder
- Salt and black pepper to taste

DIRECTIONS:

1. In a bowl, mix olive oil with salt, pepper and oil and whisk well. Brush pork shoulder with this mix, arrange in a baking dish and place in the oven at 425 degrees for 20 minutes.

2. Reduce heat to 325 degrees F and bake for 4 hours. Take pork shoulder out of the oven, slice and arrange on a platter. Serve with your favorite Mediterranean side salad.

NUTRITION: Calories 224 Fat 31g Carbs 21g Protein 23g

53. Herb Roasted Pork

Preparation time: 20 minutes

Cooking time: 2 hours

Servings: 10

INGREDIENTS:

- 5 and ½ pounds pork loin roast, trimmed, chine bone removed
- Salt and black pepper to taste
- 3 garlic cloves, minced
- 2 tablespoons rosemary, chopped
- 1 teaspoon fennel, ground
- 1 tablespoon fennel seeds
- 2 teaspoons red pepper, crushed
- ¼ cup olive oil

DIRECTIONS:

1. In a food processor mix garlic with fennel seeds, fennel, rosemary, red pepper, some black pepper and the olive oil and blend until you obtain a paste.
2. Place pork roast in a roasting pan, spread 2 tablespoons garlic paste all over and rub well. Season with salt and pepper, place in the oven at 400 degrees F and bake for 1 hour.
3. Reduce heat to 325 degrees F and bake for another 35 minutes. Carve roast into chops, divide between plates and serve right away.

NUTRITION: Calories 320 Fat 31g Carbs 21g Protein 23g

54. Slow Cooked Beef Brisket

Preparation time: 10 minutes

Cooking time: 9 hours

Servings: 8

INGREDIENTS:

- 6 pounds beef brisket
- 2 tablespoons cumin, ground
- 3 tablespoons rosemary, chopped
- 2 tablespoons coriander, dried
- 1 tablespoon oregano, dried
- 2 teaspoons cinnamon powder
- 1 cup beef stock
- A pinch of salt and black pepper

DIRECTIONS:

1. In a slow cooker, combine the beef with the cumin, rosemary, coriander, oregano, cinnamon, salt, pepper and stock. Cover and cook on low for 9 hours. Slice and serve.

NUTRITION: Calories 400 Fat 31g Carbs 21g Protein 23g

55. Mediterranean Beef Dish

Preparation time: 10 minutes

Cooking time: 15 minutes

Servings: 6

INGREDIENTS:

- 1-pound beef, ground
- 2 cups zucchinis, chopped
- ½ cup yellow onion, chopped
- Salt and black pepper to taste

- 15 ounces canned roasted tomatoes and garlic
- 1 cup water
- ¾ cup cheddar cheese, shredded
- 1 and ½ cups white rice

DIRECTIONS:

1. Heat a pan over medium high heat, add beef, onion, salt, pepper and zucchini, stir and cook for 7 minutes.
2. Add water, tomatoes and garlic, stir and bring to a boil. Add rice, more salt and pepper, stir, cover, take off heat and leave aside for 7 minutes. Divide between plates and serve with cheddar cheese on top.

NUTRITION: Calories 320 Fat 31g Carbs 21g Protein 23g

56. Beef Tartar

Preparation time: 10 minutes

Cooking time: 0 minutes

Servings: 1

INGREDIENTS:

- 1 shallot, chopped
- 4 ounces beef fillet, minced
- 5 small cucumbers, chopped
- 1 egg yolk
- A pinch of salt and black pepper
- 2 teaspoons mustard
- 1 tablespoon parsley, chopped

- 1 parsley spring, roughly chopped for serving

DIRECTIONS:

1. In a bowl, mix meat with shallot, egg yolk, salt, pepper, mustard, cucumbers and parsley. Stir well and arrange on a platter. Garnish with the chopped parsley spring and serve.

NUTRITION: Calories 244 Fat 31g Carbs 21g Protein 23g

57. Meatballs and Sauce

Preparation time: 5 minutes

Cooking time: 8 minutes

Servings: 4

INGREDIENTS:

- 1 egg, whisked
- 1 teaspoon cumin, ground
- 1 teaspoon allspice, ground
- ¼ cup cilantro, chopped
- A pinch of salt and black pepper
- 2 pounds beef, ground
- 1/3 cup breadcrumbs
- Vegetable oil for frying
- For the sauce:
- 1 cucumber, chopped
- 1 cup Greek yogurt
- 2 tablespoons lemon juice
- 1 tablespoon dill, chopped

DIRECTIONS:

1. In a bowl, mix the beef with the breadcrumbs, egg, cumin, allspice, cilantro, salt and pepper. Stir well and shape into medium sized meatballs. Heat a pan with oil over medium heat.

2. Add the meatballs and cook for 4 minutes each side. In a bowl, mix the yogurt with the cucumber, lemon juice and dill - whisk well. Serve the meatballs with the yogurt sauce.

NUTRITION: Calories 263 Fat 31g Carbs 21g Protein 23g

58. Rosemary Beef Chuck Roast

Preparation Time: 5 minutes

Cooking Time: 45 minutes

Servings: 5-6

INGREDIENTS:

- 3 pounds chuck beef roast
- 3 garlic cloves
- ¼ cup balsamic vinegar
- 1 sprig fresh rosemary
- 1 sprig fresh thyme
- 1 cup of water
- 1 tablespoon vegetable oil
- Salt and pepper to taste

DIRECTIONS:

1. Chop slices in the beef roast and place the garlic cloves in them. Rub the roast with the herbs, black pepper, and salt.

2. Preheat your instant pot using the sauté setting and pour the oil. When warmed, mix in the beef roast and stir-cook until browned on all sides.

3. Add the remaining ingredients; stir gently.

4. Seal tight and cook on high for 40 minutes using manual setting. Allow the pressure release naturally, about 10 minutes. Uncover and put the beef roast the serving plates, slice and serve.

NUTRITION: 542 Calories 11.2g Fat 8.7g Carbohydrates 55.2g Protein 710mg Sodium

59. Herb-Roasted Turkey Breast

Preparation Time: 15 minutes

Cooking Time: 1½ hours (plus 20 minutes to rest)

Servings: 2

INGREDIENTS:

- 2 tablespoons extra-virgin olive oil
- 4 garlic cloves, minced
- Zest of 1 lemon
- 1 tablespoon chopped fresh thyme leaves
- 1 tablespoon chopped fresh rosemary leaves
- 2 tablespoons chopped fresh Italian parsley leaves
- 1 teaspoon ground mustard
- 1 teaspoon sea salt
- ¼ teaspoon freshly ground black pepper
- 1 (6-pound) bone-in, skin-on turkey breast

- 1 cup dry white wine

DIRECTIONS:

1. Preheat the oven to 325°F. Combine the olive oil, garlic, lemon zest, thyme, rosemary, parsley, mustard, sea salt, and pepper.

2. Brush the herb mixture evenly over the surface of the turkey breast, and loosen the skin and rub underneath as well. Situate the turkey breast in a roasting pan on a rack, skin-side up.

3. Pour the wine in the pan. Roast for 1 to 1½ hours until the turkey reaches an internal temperature of 165 degrees F.

4. Pull out from the oven and set separately for 20 minutes, tented with aluminum foil to keep it warm, before carving.

NUTRITION: 392 Calories 1g Fat 2g Carbohydrates 84g Protein 741mg Sodium

60. Chicken Sausage and Peppers

Preparation Time: 10 minutes

Cooking Time: 20 minutes

Servings: 2

INGREDIENTS:

- 2 tablespoons extra-virgin olive oil
- 6 Italian chicken sausage links
- 1 onion
- 1 red bell pepper
- 1 green bell pepper
- 3 garlic cloves, minced

- ½ cup dry white wine
- ½ teaspoon sea salt
- ¼ teaspoon freshly ground black pepper
- Pinch red pepper flakes

DIRECTIONS:

1. Cook the olive oil on large skillet until it shimmers. Add the sausages and cook for 5 to 7 minutes, turning occasionally, until browned, and they reach an internal temperature of 165°F.
2. With tongs, remove the sausage from the pan and set aside on a platter, tented with aluminum foil to keep warm.
3. Return the skillet to the heat and mix in the onion, red bell pepper, and green bell pepper. Cook and stir occasionally, until the vegetables begin to brown.
4. Put in the garlic and cook for 30 seconds, stirring constantly.
5. Stir in the wine, sea salt, pepper, and red pepper flakes. Pull out and fold in any browned bits from the bottom of the pan.
6. Simmer for about 4 minutes more, stirring, until the liquid reduces by half. Spoon the peppers over the sausages and serve.

NUTRITION: 173 Calories 1g Fat 6g Carbohydrates 22g Protein 582mg Sodium

61. Chicken Piccata

Preparation Time: 10 minutes

Cooking Time: 15 minutes

Servings: 2

INGREDIENTS:

- ½ cup whole-wheat flour
- ½ teaspoon sea salt
- 1/8 teaspoon freshly ground black pepper
- 1½ pounds chicken breasts, cut into 6 pieces
- 3 tablespoons extra-virgin olive oil
- 1 cup unsalted chicken broth
- ½ cup dry white wine
- Juice of 1 lemon
- Zest of 1 lemon
- ¼ cup capers, drained and rinsed
- ¼ cup chopped fresh parsley leaves

DIRECTIONS:

1. In a shallow dish, whisk the flour, sea salt, and pepper. Scour the chicken in the flour and tap off any excess. Cook the olive oil until it shimmers.

2. Put the chicken and cook for about 4 minutes per side until browned. Pull out the chicken from the pan and set aside, tented with aluminum foil to keep warm.

3. Situate the skillet back to the heat and stir in the broth, wine, lemon juice, lemon zest, and capers. Use the side of a spoon scoop and fold in any browned bits from the pan's bottom.

4. Simmer until the liquid thickens. Take out the skillet from the heat and take the chicken back to the pan. Turn to coat. Stir in the parsley and serve.

NUTRITION: 153 Calories 2g Fat 9g Carbohydrates 8g Protein 692mg Sodium

62. Chicken with Onions, Potatoes, Figs, and Carrots

Preparation Time: 5 minutes

Cooking Time: 45 minutes

Servings: 2

INGREDIENTS:

- 2 cups fingerling potatoes, halved
- 4 fresh figs, quartered
- 2 carrots, julienned
- 2 tablespoons extra-virgin olive oil
- 1 teaspoon sea salt, divided
- ¼ teaspoon freshly ground black pepper
- 4 chicken leg-thigh quarters
- 2 tablespoons chopped fresh parsley leaves

DIRECTIONS:

1. Preheat the oven to 425°F. In a small bowl, toss the potatoes, figs, and carrots with the olive oil, ½ teaspoon of sea salt, and the pepper. Spread in a 9-by-13-inch baking dish.

2. Season the chicken with the rest of t sea salt. Place it on top of the vegetables. Bake until the vegetables are soft and the chicken reaches an internal temperature of 165°F.

3. Sprinkle with the parsley and serve.

NUTRITION: 429 Calories 4g Fat 27g Carbohydrates 52g Protein 581mg Sodium

63. Chicken Gyros with Tzatziki

Preparation Time: 15 minutes

Cooking Time: 1 hours and 20 minutes

Servings: 2

INGREDIENTS:

- 1-pound ground chicken breast
- 1 onion, grated with excess water wrung out
- 2 tablespoons dried rosemary
- 1 tablespoon dried marjoram
- 6 garlic cloves, minced
- ½ teaspoon sea salt
- ¼ teaspoon freshly ground black pepper
- Tzatziki Sauce

DIRECTIONS:

1. Preheat the oven to 350°F. Mix the chicken, onion, rosemary, marjoram, garlic, sea salt, and pepper using food processor.

2. Blend until the mixture forms a paste. Alternatively, mix these ingredients in a bowl until well combined (see preparation tip).

3. Press the mixture into a loaf pan. Bake until it reaches 165 degrees internal temperature. Take out from the oven and let rest for 20 minutes before slicing.

4. Slice the gyro and spoon the tzatziki sauce over the top.

NUTRITION: 289 Calories 1g Fat 20g Carbohydrates 50g Protein 622mg Sodium

64. Greek Chicken Salad

Preparation Time: 15 minutes

Cooking Time: 30 minutes

Servings: 2

INGREDIENTS:

- 1/4 cup balsamic vinegar
- 1 teaspoon freshly squeezed lemon juice
- 1/4 cup extra-virgin olive oil
- 1/4 teaspoon salt
- 1/4 teaspoon freshly ground black pepper
- 2 grilled boneless, skinless chicken breasts, sliced (about 1 cup)

- 1/2 cup thinly sliced red onion
- 10 cherry tomatoes, halved
- 8 pitted Kalamata olives, halved
- 2 cups roughly chopped romaine lettuce
- 1/2 cup feta cheese

DIRECTIONS:

1. In a medium bowl, combine the vinegar and lemon juice and stir well. Slowly whisk in the olive oil and continue whisking vigorously until well blended. Whisk in the salt and pepper.

2. Add the chicken, onion, tomatoes, and olives and stir well. Cover and refrigerate for at least 2 hours or overnight.

3. To serve, divide the romaine between 2 salad plates and top each with half of the chicken vegetable mixture. Top with feta cheese and serve immediately.

NUTRITION: 173 Calories 1g Fat 6g Carbohydrates 22g Protein 582mg Sodium

65. One Pot Greek Chicken and Lemon Rice

Preparation Time: 15 minutes

Cooking Time: 30 minutes

Servings: 20

INGREDIENTS:

- Chicken and Marinade
- 5 chicken thighs, skin on, bone in (about 1 kg / 2 lb.) (Note 1)
- 1 - 2 lemons, use the zest + 4 tbsp lemon juice (Note 7)
- 1 tbsp dried oregano
- 4 garlic cloves, minced
- 1/2 tsp salt
- Rice
- 1 1/2 tbsp olive oil, separated
- 1 small onion, finely diced
- 1 cup (180g) long grain rice, uncooked (Note 6)
- 1 1/2 cups (375 ml) chicken broth / stock
- 3/4 cup (185 ml) water

- 1 tbsp dried oregano
- 3/4 tsp salt
- Black pepper
- Garnish
- Finely chopped parsley or oregano (optional)
- Fresh lemon zest (highly recommended)

DIRECTIONS:

1. Combine the Chicken and Marinade ingredients in a Ziplock bag and set aside for at least 20 minutes but preferably overnight.
2. TO COOK
3. Preheat oven to 180°C/350°F.
4. Remove chicken from marinade, but reserve the Marinade.
5. Heat 1/2 tbsp olive oil in a deep, heavy based skillet (Note 2) over medium high heat.
6. Place the chicken in the skillet, skin side down, and cook until golden brown, then turn and cook the other side until golden brown.
7. Remove the chicken and set aside.
8. Pour off fat and wipe the pan with a scrunched-up ball of paper towel (to remove black bits), then return to the stove.
9. Heat 1 tbsp olive oil in the skillet over medium high heat. Add the onion and sauté for a few minutes until translucent.
10. Then add the remaining Rice ingredients and reserved Marinade.
11. Let the liquid come to a simmer and let it simmer for 30 seconds. Place the chicken on top then place a lid on the skillet (Note 3).

12. Bake in the oven for 35 minutes. Then remove the lid and bake for a further 10 minutes, or until all the liquid is absorbed and the rice is tender (so 45 minutes in total).

13. Remove from the oven and allow to rest for 5 to 10 minutes before serving, garnished with parsley or oregano and fresh lemon zest, if desired.

NUTRITION: 173 Calories 1g Fat 6g Carbohydrates 22g Protein 582mg Sodium

66. **Balsamic Beef Dish**

Preparation Time: 15 minutes

Cooking Time: 45 minutes

Servings: 2

INGREDIENTS:

- 3 lbs. or 1360 g chuck roast
- 3 cloves garlic, sliced
- 1 tbsp. oil
- 1 tsp. flavored vinegar
- ½ tsp. pepper
- ½ tsp. rosemary
- 1 tbsp. butter
- ½ tsp. thyme
- 1 c. beef broth

DIRECTIONS:

1. Slice-slit openings in the roast and stuff them with garlic slices.

2. Using a bowl, combine pepper, vinegar, and rosemary. Rub all over the roast.

3. Place your pot on heat. Add in oil and heat on sauté mode.

4. Add in the roast and cook until both sides brown (each side to take 5 minutes). Remove from pot and set aside.

5. Add in thyme, broth, butter, and deglaze your pot.

6. Set back the roast and cook for 40 minutes on High heat while covered.

7. Remove the lid and serve!

NUTRITION: Calories 393, Fat 15 g, Sat. fat 6 g, Fiber 11 g, Carbs 25 g, Sugars 8 g, Protein 37 g, Sodium 438mg

67. Greek Chicken with Vegetables and Lemon Vinaigrette

Preparation Time: 15 minutes

Cooking Time: 50 minutes

Servings: 2

INGREDIENTS:

- For the lemon vinaigrette
- 1 tsp. lemon zest
- 1 tbsp. lemon juice
- 1 tbsp. olive oil
- 1 tbsp. crumbled feta cheese
- ½ tsp. honey
- For the Greek Chicken and roasted veggies

- 8 oz. or 226.7g boneless chicken breast, skinless and halved
- ¼ c. light mayonnaise
- 2 cloves minced garlic
- ½ c. panko bread crumbs
- 3 tbsps. Parmesan cheese, grated
- ½ tsp. kosher salt
- ½ tsp. black pepper
- 1 tbsp. olive oil
- ½ c. dill sliced

DIRECTIONS:

1. To make the vinaigrette, put a teaspoon of zest, one tablespoon of lemon juice, olive oil, cheese, and honey in a bowl.

2. For the vegetables and chicken, preheat the oven to 470 F/243 C. Use a meat mallet for flattening the chicken to two pieces.

3. Using a bowl, set in the chicken. Add in two garlic cloves and mayonnaise. Mix cheese, bread crumbs, pepper, and salt together. Dip the chicken in this crumb mix. Spray olive oil over the chicken.

4. Roast in the oven till the chicken is done and vegetables are tender. Sprinkle dill over it and serve.

NUTRITION: Calories 306, Fat 15 g, Sat. fat 3 g, Fiber 2 g, Carbs 12 g, Sugar 4 g, Protein 30 g, Sodium 432 mg

68. Simple Grilled Salmon with Veggies

Preparation Time: 10 minutes

Cooking Time: 25 minutes

Servings: 2

INGREDIENTS:

- 1 halved zucchini
- 2 trimmed oranges, red or yellow bell peppers, halved and seeded
- 1 red onion, wedged
- 1 tbsp. olive oil
- ½ tsp. salt and ground pepper
- 1¼ lbs. or 0.57kg salmon fillet, 4 slices
- ¼ c. sliced fresh basil
- 1 lemon, wedged

DIRECTIONS:

1. Preheat the grill to medium-high. Brush peppers, zucchini, and onion with oil. Sprinkle a ¼ teaspoon of salt over it. Sprinkle salmon with salt and pepper.

2. Place the veggies and the salmon on the grill. Cook the veggies for six to eight minutes on each side, till the grill marks appear. Cook the salmon till it flakes when you test it with a fork.

3. When cooled down, chop the veggies roughly and mix them in a bowl. You can remove the salmon skin to serve with the veggies.

4. Each serving can be garnished with a tablespoon of basil and a lemon wedge.

NUTRITION: Calories 281, Fat 13 g, Sat. fat 2 g, Fiber 6 g, Carbs 11 g, Sugars 6 g, Protein 30 g, Sodium 369 mg

69. Caprese Chicken Hasselback Style

Preparation Time: 10 minutes

Cooking Time: 30 minutes

Servings: 2

INGREDIENTS:

- 2 (8 oz. or 226.7g each) skinless chicken breasts, boneless
- ½ tsp. salt
- ½ tsp. ground pepper
- 1 sliced tomato
- 3 oz. or 85g fresh mozzarella, halved and sliced
- ¼ c. prepared pesto
- 8 c. broccoli florets
- 2 tbsps. olive oil

DIRECTIONS:

1. Set your oven to 375 F/190 C and coat a rimmed baking sheet with cooking spray.
2. Make crosswire cuts at half inches in the chicken breasts. Sprinkle ¼ teaspoons of pepper and salt on them. Fill the cuts with mozzarella slices and tomato alternatively. Brush both the chicken breasts with pesto and put it on the baking sheet.
3. Mix broccoli, oil, salt, and pepper in a bowl. Put this mixture on one side of the baking sheet.
4. Bake till the broccoli is tender, and the chicken is not pink in the center. Cut each of the breasts in half and serve.

NUTRITION: Calories 355 Fat 19 g, Sat. fat 6 g, Fiber 3 g, Carbs 4 g, Sugars 3 g, Protein 38 g, Sodium 634

70. Grilled Calamari with Lemon Juice

Preparation Time: 10 minutes

Cooking Time: 15 minutes

Servings: 2

INGREDIENTS:

- ¼ c. dried cranberries
- ¼ c. extra virgin olive oil
- ¼ c. olive oil
- ¼ c. sliced almonds
- 1/3 c. fresh lemon juice
- ¾ c. blueberries
- 1 ½ lbs. or 700 g. cleaned calamari tube
- 1 granny smith apple, sliced thinly
- 2 tbsps. apple cider vinegar
- 6 c. fresh spinach
- Grated pepper
- Sea salt

DIRECTIONS:

1. In a medium bowl, mix lemon juice, apple cider vinegar, and extra virgin olive oil to make a sauce. Season with pepper and salt to taste and mix well.

2. Turn on the grill to medium fire and let the grates heat up for 1-2 minutes.

3. In a separate bowl, add in olive oil and the calamari tube. Season calamari generously with pepper and salt.

4. Place calamari onto heated grate and grill for 2-3 minutes each side or until opaque.

5. Meanwhile, combine almonds, cranberries, blueberries, spinach, and the thinly sliced apple in a large salad bowl. Toss to mix.

6. Remove cooked calamari from grill and transfer on a chopping board. Cut into ¼-inch thick rings and throw into the salad bowl.

7. Sprinkle with already prepared sauce. Toss well to coat and serve.

NUTRITION: Calories 567, Fat 24 g, Sat. fat 5 g, Fiber 2 g, Carbs 30.6 g, Sugars 1 g, Protein 54.8 g, Sodium 320 mg

71. Bacon-Wrapped Chicken

Preparation Time: 10 minutes

Cooking Time: 50 minutes

Servings: 2

INGREDIENTS:

- 4 slices Bacon
- Salt
- Pepper
- 4 oz. or 113 g. Cheddar Cheese, grated
- 2 Chicken Breasts

- Paprika to taste
- 2 tbsps. lemon or orange fresh juice

DIRECTIONS:

1. Heat the oven to 350 F/ 176 C.
2. Place chicken breasts into a medium bowl and season with salt, pepper, paprika, and fresh juice.
3. Replace chicken breasts to a baking pan.
4. Add cheese on top and place bacon slices over chicken breasts.
5. Place the baking pan to the oven for 45 minutes.
6. Take away from the oven your dish and the double-meat meal are ready to be served.
7. Note: If you want to get extra crispy bacon, place your cooked breasts covered with cheese and bacon on a grill or skillet and sauté for 2 minutes on each side.

NUTRITION: Calories 206, Fat 8 g, Sat. fat 3.7 g, Fiber 0 g, Carbs 1.6 g, Sugars 1.6 g, Protein 30 g, Sodium 302 mg

72. Broccoli Pesto Spaghetti

Preparation Time: 10 minutes

Cooking Time: 20 minutes

Servings: 2

INGREDIENTS:

- 8 oz. or 226.7g spaghetti
- 1 lb. or 450g broccoli, cut into florets
- 2 tbsps. olive oil
- 4 garlic cloves, chopped

- 4 basil leaves

- 2 tbsps. blanched almonds

- 1 juiced lemon

- Salt and pepper

DIRECTIONS:

1. For the pesto, combine the broccoli, oil, garlic, basil, lemon juice and almonds in a blender and pulse until well mixed and smooth.

2. Set spaghetti in a pot, add salt and pepper. Cook until al dente for about 8 minutes. Drain well.

3. Mix the warm spaghetti with the broccoli pesto and serve.

NUTRITION: Calories 284, Fat 10.2 g, Sat. fat 3 g, Fiber 10 g, Carbs 40.2 g, Sugar 6 g, Protein 10.4 g, Sodium 421 mg

MAIN RECIPES: SEAFOOD

73. Classic Escabeche

Preparation time: 15 minutes

Cooking time: 20 minutes

Servings: 4

INGREDIENTS:

- 1 pound (454 g) wild-caught Spanish mackerel fillets, cut into four pieces
- 1 teaspoon salt
- ½ teaspoon freshly ground black pepper
- 8 tablespoons extra-virgin olive oil, divided
- 1 bunch asparagus, trimmed and cut into 2-inch pieces
- 1 (13¾-ounce / 390-g) can artichoke hearts, drained and quartered
- 4 large garlic cloves, peeled and crushed
- 2 bay leaves
- ¼ cup red wine vinegar
- ½ teaspoon smoked paprika

DIRECTIONS:

1. Sprinkle the fillets with salt and pepper and let sit at room temperature for 5 minutes.

2. In a large skillet, heat 2 tablespoons olive oil over medium-high heat. Add the fish, skin-side up, and cook 5 minutes.

3. Flip and cook 5 minutes on the other side, until browned and cooked through. Transfer to a serving dish, pour the cooking oil over the fish, and cover to keep warm.

4. Heat the remaining 6 tablespoons olive oil in the same skillet over medium heat. Add the asparagus, artichokes, garlic, and bay leaves and sauté until the vegetables are tender, 6 to 8 minutes.

5. Using a slotted spoon, top the fish with the cooked vegetables, reserving the oil in the skillet. Add the vinegar and paprika to the oil and whisk to combine well.

6. Pour the vinaigrette over the fish and vegetables and let sit at room temperature for at least 15 minutes, or marinate in the refrigerator up to 24 hours for a deeper flavor. Remove the bay leaf before serving.

NUTRITION: Calories: 578 Fat: 50g Protein: 26g Carbs: 13g

74. Olive Oil-Poached Tuna

Preparation time: 15 minutes

Cooking time: 45 minutes

Servings: 4

INGREDIENTS:

- 1 cup extra-virgin olive oil, plus more if needed
- 4 (3- to 4-inch) sprigs fresh rosemary
- 8 (3- to 4-inch) sprigs fresh thyme
- 2 large garlic cloves, thinly sliced

- 2 (2-inch) strips lemon zest
- 1 teaspoon salt
- ½ teaspoon freshly ground black pepper
- 1 pound (454 g) fresh tuna steaks (about 1 inch thick)

DIRECTIONS:

1. Select a thick pot just large enough to fit the tuna in a single layer on the bottom. The larger the pot, the more olive oil you will need to use.

2. Combine the olive oil, rosemary, thyme, garlic, lemon zest, salt, and pepper over medium-low heat and cook until warm and fragrant, 20 to 25 minutes, lowering the heat if it begins to smoke.

3. Remove from the heat and allow to cool for 25 to 30 minutes, until warm but not hot.

4. Add the tuna to the bottom of the pan, adding additional oil if needed so that tuna is fully submerged, and return to medium-low heat.

5. Cook for 5 to 10 minutes, or until the oil heats back up and is warm and fragrant but not smoking. Lower the heat if it gets too hot.

6. Remove the pot from the heat and let the tuna cook in warm oil 4 to 5 minutes, to your desired level of doneness. For a tuna that is rare in the center, cook for 2 to 3 minutes.

7. Remove from the oil and serve warm, drizzling 2 to 3 tablespoons seasoned oil over the tuna.

8. To store for later use, remove the tuna from the oil and place in a container with a lid. Allow tuna and oil to cool separately.

9. When both have cooled, remove the herb stems with a slotted spoon and pour the cooking oil over the tuna.

10. Cover and store in the refrigerator for up to 1 week. Bring to room temperature to allow the oil to liquify before serving.

NUTRITION: Calories: 363 Fat: 28g Protein: 27g Carbs: 1g

75. <u>Fideos with Seafood</u>

Preparation time: 15 minutes

Cooking time: 20 minutes

Servings: 6-8

INGREDIENTS:

- 2 tablespoons extra-virgin olive oil, plus ½ cup, divided
- 6 cups zucchini noodles, roughly chopped (2 to 3 medium zucchini)
- 1 pound (454 g) shrimp, peeled, deveined and roughly chopped
- 6 to 8 ounces (170 to 227 g) canned chopped clams, drained
- 4 ounces (113 g) crab meat
- ½ cup crumbled goat cheese
- ½ cup crumbled feta cheese
- 1 (28-ounce / 794-g) can chopped tomatoes, with their juices
- 1 teaspoon salt
- 1 teaspoon garlic powder
- ½ teaspoon smoked paprika

- ½ cup shredded Parmesan cheese
- ¼ cup chopped fresh flat-leaf Italian parsley, for garnish

DIRECTIONS:

1. Preheat the oven to 375°F (190°C). Pour 2 tablespoons olive oil in the bottom of a 9-by-13-inch baking dish and swirl to coat the bottom.

2. In a large bowl, combine the zucchini noodles, shrimp, clams, and crab meat. In another bowl, combine the goat cheese, feta, and ¼ cup olive oil and stir to combine well.

3. Add the canned tomatoes and their juices, salt, garlic powder, and paprika and combine well. Add the mixture to the zucchini and seafood mixture and stir to combine.

4. Pour the mixture into the prepared baking dish, spreading evenly. Spread shredded Parmesan over top and drizzle with the remaining ¼ cup olive oil.

5. Bake until bubbly, 20 to 25 minutes. Serve warm, garnished with chopped parsley.

NUTRITION: Calories: 434 Fat: 31g Protein: 29g Carbs: 12g

76. Shrimp Pesto Rice Bowls

Preparation time: 5 minutes

Cooking time: 5 minutes

Servings: 4

INGREDIENTS:

- 1 pound (454 g) medium shrimp, peeled and deveined
- ¼ cup pesto sauce

- 1 lemon, sliced
- 2 cups cooked wild rice pilaf

DIRECTIONS:

1. Preheat the air fryer to 360°F (182°C). In a medium bowl, toss the shrimp with the pesto sauce until well coated.
2. Place the shrimp in a single layer in the air fryer basket. Put the lemon slices over the shrimp and roast for 5 minutes.
3. Remove the lemons and discard. Serve a quarter of the shrimp over ½ cup wild rice with some favorite steamed vegetables.

NUTRITION: Calories: 249 Fat: 10g Protein: 20g Carbs: 20g

77. Salmon with Tomatoes and Olives

Preparation time: 5 minutes

Cooking time: 8 minutes

Servings: 4

INGREDIENTS:

- 2 tablespoons olive oil
- 4 (1½-inch-thick) salmon fillets
- ½ teaspoon salt
- ¼ teaspoon cayenne
- 1 teaspoon chopped fresh dill
- 2 Roma tomatoes, diced
- ¼ cup sliced Kalamata olives
- 4 lemon slices

DIRECTIONS:

1. Preheat the air fryer to 380°F (193°C). Brush the olive oil on both sides of the salmon fillets, and then season them lightly with salt, cayenne, and dill.

2. Place the fillets in a single layer in the basket of the air fryer, then layer the tomatoes and olives over the top. Top each fillet with a lemon slice.

3. Bake for 8 minutes, or until the salmon has reached an internal temperature of 145°F (63°C).

NUTRITION: Calories: 241 Fat: 15g Protein: 23g Carbs: 3g

78. Baked Trout with Lemon

Preparation time: 5 minutes

Cooking time: 15 minutes

Servings: 4

INGREDIENTS:

- 4 trout fillets
- 2 tablespoons olive oil
- ½ teaspoon salt
- 1 teaspoon black pepper
- 2 garlic cloves, sliced
- 1 lemon, sliced, plus additional wedges for serving

DIRECTIONS:

1. Preheat the air fryer to 380°F (193°C). Brush each fillet with olive oil on both sides and season with salt and pepper. Place the fillets in an even layer in the air fryer basket.

2. Place the sliced garlic over the tops of the trout fillets, then top the garlic with lemon slices and cook for 12 to 15 minutes. Serve with fresh lemon wedges.

NUTRITION: Calories: 231 Fat: 12g Protein: 29g Carbs: 1g

79. Shrimp and Pea Paella

Preparation Time: 20 minutes

Cooking Time: 60 minutes

Serving: 2

INGREDIENTS:

- 2 tablespoons olive oil
- 1 garlic clove, minced
- ½ large onion, minced
- 1 cup diced tomato
- ½ cup short-grain rice
- ½ teaspoon sweet paprika
- ½ cup dry white wine
- 1¼ cups low-sodium chicken stock
- 8 ounces (227 g) large raw shrimp
- 1 cup frozen peas
- ¼ cup jarred roasted red peppers

DIRECTION

1. Heat the olive oil in a large skillet over medium-high heat.
2. Add the garlic and onion and sauté for 3 minutes, or until the onion is softened.

3. Add the tomato, rice, and paprika and stir for 3 minutes to toast the rice.

4. Add the wine and chicken stock and stir to combine. Bring the mixture to a boil.

5. Cover and set heat to medium-low, and simmer for 45 minutes

6. Add the shrimp, peas, and roasted red peppers. Cover and cook for an additional 5 minutes. Season with salt to taste and serve.

NUTRITION: Calories 646, 27g fat, 42g protein

80. Garlic Shrimp with Arugula Pesto

Preparation Time: 20 minutes

Cooking Time: 5 minutes

Serving: 2

INGREDIENTS:

- 3 cups lightly packed arugula
- ½ cup lightly packed basil leaves
- ¼ cup walnuts
- 3 tablespoons olive oil
- 3 medium garlic cloves
- 2 tablespoons grated Parmesan cheese
- 1 tablespoon freshly squeezed lemon juice
- 1 (10-ounce) package zucchini noodles
- 8 ounces (227 g) cooked, shelled shrimp
- 2 Roma tomatoes, diced

DIRECTION

1. Process the arugula, basil, walnuts, olive oil, garlic, Parmesan cheese, and lemon juice in a food processor until smooth, scraping down the sides as needed. Season

2. Heat a skillet over medium heat. Add the pesto, zucchini noodles, and cooked shrimp. Toss to combine the sauce over the noodles and shrimp, and cook until heated through.

3. Season well. Serve topped with the diced tomatoes.

NUTRITION: Calories 435, 30.2g fat, 33g protein

81. Baked Oysters with Vegetables

Preparation Time: 30 minutes

Cooking Time: 17 minutes

Serving: 2

INGREDIENTS:

- 2 cups coarse salt, for holding the oysters
- 1 dozen fresh oysters, scrubbed
- 1 tablespoon almond butter
- ¼ cup finely chopped scallions
- ½ cup finely chopped artichoke hearts
- ¼ cup finely chopped red bell pepper
- 1 garlic clove, minced
- 1 tablespoon finely chopped fresh parsley
- Zest and juice of ½ lemon

DIRECTION:

1. Pour the salt into a baking dish and spread to fill the bottom of the dish evenly.

2. Using a shucking knife, insert the blade at the joint of the shell, where it hinges open and shut. Firmly apply pressure to pop the blade in, and work the knife around the shell to open. Discard the empty half of the shell. Using the knife, gently loosen the oyster, and remove any shell particles. Sprinkle salt in the oysters

3. Set oven to 425°F (220°C).

4. Heat the almond butter in a large skillet over medium heat. Add the scallions, artichoke hearts, and bell pepper, and cook for 5 to 7 minutes. Cook garlic

5. Takeout from the heat and stir in the parsley, lemon zest and juice, and season to taste with salt and pepper.

6. Divide the vegetable mixture evenly among the oysters. Bake in the preheated oven for 10 to 12 minutes.

NUTRITION: Calories 135, 7g fat, 6g protein

82. Creamy Fish Gratin

Preparation Time: 10 minutes

Cooking Time: 55 minutes

Serving: 6

INGREDIENTS:

- 1 c. heavy cream
- 2 cubed salmon fillets
- 2 cod fillets, cubed
- 2 sea bass fillets, cubed

- 1 celery stalk, sliced
- Salt and pepper
- ½ c. grated Parmesan
- ½ c. crumbled feta cheese

DIRECTIONS:

1. Combine the cream with the fish fillets and celery in a deep-dish baking pan.
2. Add salt and pepper to taste then top with the Parmesan and feta cheese.
3. Cook in the preheated oven at 350 F/176 C for 20 minutes.
4. Serve the gratin and enjoy it.

NUTRITION: Calories 301, Fat 16.1 g, Sat. fat 5 g, Fiber 0.2 g, Carbs 1.3 g, Sugar 0 g, Protein 36.9 g, Sodium 211 mg

83. Mixed Seafood Dish

Preparation Time: 10 minutes

Cooking Time: 35 minutes

Serving: 4

INGREDIENTS:

- 12 scrubbed clams, cleaned
- 3 chopped dried chilies, soaked and drained
- 1 lobster, tail separated and halved
- 1 c. water
- ¼ c. flour
- 3 tbsps. olive oil

- 1 ½ lbs. or 700 g. skinless monkfish, boneless and thinly sliced into fillets
- Salt and black pepper
- 35 unpeeled shrimp
- 1 chopped onion
- 4 minced garlic cloves
- 4 grated tomatoes
- 1 baguette slice, toasted
- 30 skinned hazelnuts
- 2 tbsps. chopped parsley
- 1 c. fish stock
- ¼ tsp. smoked paprika
- Lemon wedges
- Crusty bread slices

DIRECTIONS:

1. Put the water in a large saucepan, bring to a boil over high heat
2. Add clams, cover and cook for 4 minutes. Take away from heat and discard unopened ones.
3. Heat a skillet with olive oil over medium-high heat.
4. Meantime, put flour on a medium bowl and dredge in fish.
5. Season with salt and pepper.
6. Place fish into the skillet and cook for 3 minutes on each side, after transfer to a plate
7. Add shrimps to the same skillet and cook for about 2 minutes on each side, transfer to a plate.

8. Reduce heat to medium-low, add garlic to the same pan, stir, cook for 1 minute and transfer to a blender.

9. Add onion to the skillet and stir for 3 minutes.

10. Add tomatoes, stir and cook on a low heat for 7 minutes.

NUTRITION: Calories 344, 18g fat, 21g protein

SNACK RECIPES

84. Watermelon Feta & Balsamic Pizza

Preparation Time: 5 minutes

Cooking Time: 15 minutes

Servings: 4

INGREDIENTS:

- Watermelon (1-inch thick from the center)
- Crumbled feta cheese (1 oz.)
- Sliced Kalamata olives (5-6)
- Mint leaves (1 tsp.)
- Balsamic glaze (.5 tbsp.)

DIRECTIONS:

1. Slice the widest section of the watermelon in half. Then, slice each half into four wedges. Serve on a round pie dish like a pizza round and cover with the olives, cheese, mint leaves, and glaze.

NUTRITION: Calories: 90 Protein: 2 g Fat: 3 g Carbs 5 g

85. Tomato and Cherry Linguine

Preparation Time: 10 Minutes

Cooking Time: 15 Minutes

Servings: 4

INGREDIENTS:

- 2 pounds cherry tomatoes
- 3 tablespoons extra virgin olive oil
- 2 tablespoons balsamic vinegar
- 2 teaspoons garlic, minced
- Pinch of fresh ground black pepper
- ¾ pound whole-wheat linguine pasta
- 1 tablespoon fresh oregano, chopped
- ¼ cup feta cheese, crumbled

DIRECTIONS:

1. Pre-heat your oven to 350 degrees Fahrenheit.
2. Take a large bowl and add cherry tomatoes, 2 tablespoons olive oil, balsamic vinegar, garlic, pepper and toss.
3. Spread tomatoes evenly on baking sheet and roast for 15 minutes.
4. While the tomatoes are roasting, cook the pasta according to the package instructions and drain the paste into a large bowl.
5. Toss pasta with 1 tablespoon olive oil.
6. Add roasted tomatoes (with juice) and toss.
7. Serve with topping of oregano and feta cheese.
8. Enjoy!

NUTRITION: Calories: 397 Fat: 15g Carbohydrates: 55g Protein: 13g

86. Mediterranean Zucchini Mushroom Pasta

Preparation Time: 10 Minutes

Cooking Time: 10 Minutes

Servings: 4

INGREDIENTS:

- ½ pound pasta
- 2 tablespoons olive oil
- 6 garlic cloves, crushed
- 1 teaspoon red chili
- 2 spring onions, sliced
- 3 teaspoons rosemary
- 1 large zucchini, cut in half
- 5 large portabella mushrooms
- 1 can tomatoes
- 4 tablespoons Parmesan cheese
- Fresh ground black pepper

DIRECTIONS:

1. Cook the pasta.
2. Take a large-sized frying pan and place it over medium heat.
3. Add oil and allow the oil to heat up.
4. Add garlic, onion and chili and sauté for a few minutes until golden.

5. Add zucchini, rosemary and mushroom and sauté for a few minutes.

6. Increase the heat to medium-high and add tinned tomatoes to the sauce until thick.

7. Drain your boiled pasta and transfer to serving platter.

8. Pour the tomato mix on top and mix using tongs.

9. Garnish with Parmesan and freshly ground black pepper.

10. Enjoy!

NUTRITION: Calories: 361 Fat: 12g Carbohydrates: 47g Protein: 14g

87. Lemon and Garlic Fettucine

Preparation Time: 5 Minutes

Cooking Time: 15 Minutes

Servings: 5

INGREDIENTS:

- 8 ounces of whole wheat fettuccine
- 4 tablespoons of extra virgin olive oil
- 4 cloves of minced garlic
- 1 cup of fresh breadcrumbs
- ¼ cup of lemon juice
- 1 teaspoon of freshly ground pepper
- ½ teaspoon of salt
- 2 cans of 4 ounce boneless and skinless sardines (dipped in tomato sauce)
- ½ cup of chopped up fresh parsley

- ¼ cup of finely shredded Parmesan cheese

DIRECTIONS:

1. Take a large-sized pot and bring water to a boil.
2. Cook pasta for 10 minutes until Al Dente.
3. Take a small-sized skillet and place it over medium heat.
4. Add 2 tablespoons of oil and allow it to heat up.
5. Add garlic and cook for 20 seconds.
6. Transfer the garlic to a medium-sized bowl
7. Add breadcrumbs to the hot skillet and cook for 5-6 minutes until golden
8. Whisk in lemon juice, pepper and salt into the garlic bowl
9. Add pasta to the bowl (with garlic) and sardines, parsley and Parmesan
10. Stir well and sprinkle bread crumbs
11. Enjoy!

NUTRITION: Calories: 480 Fat: 21g Carbohydrates: 53g Protein: 23g

88. Roasted Broccoli with Parmesan

Preparation Time: 10 Minutes

Cooking Time: 10 Minutes

Servings: 4

INGREDIENTS:

- 2 head broccolis, cut into florets
- 2 tablespoons extra-virgin olive oil
- 2 teaspoons garlic, minced
- Zest of 1 lemon

- Pinch of salt
- ½ cup Parmesan cheese, grated

DIRECTIONS:

1. Pre-heat your oven to 400 degrees Fahrenheit.
2. Take a large bowl and add broccoli with 2 tablespoons olive oil, lemon zest, garlic, lemon juice and salt.
3. Spread mix on the baking sheet in single layer and sprinkle with Parmesan cheese.
4. Bake for 10 minutes until tender.
5. Transfer broccoli to serving the dish.
6. Serve and enjoy!

NUTRITION: Calories: 154 Fat: 11g Carbohydrates: 10g Protein: 9g

89. Spinach and Feta Bread

Preparation Time: 10 Minutes

Cooking Time: 12 Minutes

Servings: 6

INGREDIENTS:

- 6 ounces of sun-dried tomato pesto
- 6 pieces of 6-inch whole wheat pita bread
- 2 chopped up Roma plum tomatoes
- 1 bunch of rinsed and chopped spinach
- 4 sliced fresh mushrooms
- ½ cup of crumbled feta cheese
- 2 tablespoons of grated Parmesan cheese

- 3 tablespoons of olive oil
- Ground black pepper as needed

DIRECTIONS:

1. Pre-heat your oven to 350 degrees Fahrenheit.
2. Spread your tomato pesto onto one side of your pita bread and place on your baking sheet (with the pesto side up).
3. Top up the pitas with spinach, tomatoes, feta cheese, mushrooms and Parmesan cheese.
4. Drizzle with some olive oil and season nicely with pepper.
5. Bake in your oven for around 12 minutes until the breads are crispy.
6. Cut up the pita into quarters and serve!

NUTRITION: Calories: 350 Fat: 17g Carbohydrates: 41g Protein: 11g

90. Quick Zucchini Bowl

Preparation Time: 10 Minutes

Cooking Time: 10 Minutes

Servings: 4

INGREDIENTS:

- ½ pound of pasta
- 2 tablespoons of olive oil
- 6 crushed garlic cloves
- 1 teaspoon of red chili
- 2 finely sliced spring onions
- 3 teaspoons of chopped rosemary

- 1 large zucchini cut up in half, lengthways and sliced
- 5 large portabella mushrooms
- 1 can of tomatoes
- 4 tablespoons of Parmesan cheese
- Fresh ground black pepper

DIRECTIONS:

1. Cook the pasta.
2. Take a large-sized frying pan and place over medium heat.
3. Add oil and allow the oil to heat up.
4. Add garlic, onion and chili and sauté for a few minutes until golden.
5. Add zucchini, rosemary and mushroom and sauté for a few minutes.
6. Increase the heat to medium-high and add tinned tomatoes to the sauce until thick.
7. Drain your boiled pasta and transfer to a serving platter.
8. Pour the tomato mix on top and mix using tongs.
9. Garnish with Parmesan cheese and freshly ground black pepper.
10. Enjoy!

NUTRITION: Calories: 361 Fat: 12g Carbohydrates: 47g Protein: 14g

91. Healthy Basil Platter

Preparation Time: 25 Minutes

Cooking Time: 15 Minutes

Servings: 4

INGREDIENTS:

- 2 pieces of red pepper seeded and cut up into chunks
- 2 pieces of red onion cut up into wedges
- 2 mild red chilies, diced and seeded
- 3 coarsely chopped garlic cloves
- 1 teaspoon of golden caster sugar
- 2 tablespoons of olive oil (plus additional for serving)
- 2 pounds of small ripe tomatoes quartered up
- 12 ounces of dried pasta
- Just a handful of basil leaves
- 2 tablespoons of grated Parmesan

DIRECTIONS:

1. Pre-heat the oven to 392 degrees Fahrenheit.
2. Take a large-sized roasting tin and scatter pepper, red onion, garlic and chilies.
3. Sprinkle sugar on top.
4. Drizzle olive oil then season with pepper and salt.
5. Roast the veggies in your oven for 15 minutes.
6. Take a large-sized pan and cook the pasta in boiling, salted water until Al Dente.
7. Drain them.
8. Remove the veggies from the oven and tip in the pasta into the veggies.
9. Toss well and tear basil leaves on top.
10. Sprinkle Parmesan and enjoy!

NUTRITION: Calories: 452 Fat: 8g Carbohydrates: 88g Protein: 14g

92. Crispy Sweet Potato Fries

Preparation Time: 15 minutes

Cooking Time: 10 minutes

Servings: 4

INGREDIENTS

- 1 1/2 lbs. sweet potatoes

- Sea salt

- Garlic powder

- Onion powder

DIRECTIONS:

1. In a cast-iron skillet over medium-high to high heat, add 1/2 to 1 inch of oil. When the oil is hot and you can begin to see little air pockets forming, add the sweet potato fries to the container.

2. Fry until they are brilliant darker and marginally firm, around 10 minutes. Remove from oil and move to a paper towel to absorb excess oil.

3. Add sea salt, garlic powder and onion powder in a little bowl. Sprinkle flavoring over top of the sweet potato fries.

NUTRITION: Calories: 368 Carbs: 62g Fat: 14g Protein: 28g

93. Baked Eggs and Asparagus with Parmesan

Preparation Time: 7 minutes

Cooking Time: 18 minutes

Servings: 2

INGREDIENTS:

- thick asparagus spears
- 4- eggs
- 2- tsp. olive oil
- salt and black pepper
- 2 tbsp Parmesan cheese

DIRECTIONS:

1. Preheat the stove to 400F/200C and shower two gratin dishes with a spray of olive oil.

2. Break each egg into a little dish and give eggs a chance to come to room temperature while you cook the asparagus.

3. Remove the base of every asparagus and dispose of it. Cut the remainder of asparagus into short pieces under 2 inches in length.

4. Put a large portion of the asparagus pieces into each gratin dish and put dishes into the stove to cook the asparagus, setting a clock for 10 minutes.

5. Once the timer goes off, remove gratin dishes from the stove and cautiously slide two eggs over the asparagus in each dish. Set back in the stove and set the clock for 5 minutes.

6. Following 5 minutes, remove gratin dishes and sprinkle each with a tablespoon of coarsely-ground Parmesan.

NUTRITION: Calories: 394 Carbs: 4g Fat: 32g Protein: 24g

94. Flavorful Braised Kale

Preparation Time: 9 minutes

Cooking Time: 23 minutes

Servings: 6

INGREDIENTS:

- 1 lb. kale, stems removed & chopped roughly
- 1 cup cherry tomatoes, halved
- 4 cloves garlic, sliced thin
- ½ cup vegetable stock
- 1 tablespoon lemon juice, fresh

DIRECTIONS:

1. Warm up olive oil in a frying pan using medium heat, and add in your garlic. Sauté for a minute or two until lightly golden. Mix your kale and vegetable stock with your garlic, adding it to your pan.

2. Cover the pan and then turn the heat down to medium-low. Allow it to cook until your kale wilts and part of your vegetable stock should be dissolved. It should take roughly five minutes.

3. Stir in your tomatoes and cook without a lid until your kale is tender, and then remove it from heat. Mix in your salt, pepper and lemon juice before serving warm.

NUTRITION: Calories: 100 Carbs: 8g Fat: 7g Protein: 3g

95. Basil Tomato Skewers

Preparation Time: 6 minutes

Cooking Time: 0 minute

Servings: 2

INGREDIENTS:

- 16 mozzarella balls, fresh & small
- 16 basil leaves, fresh
- 16 cherry tomatoes
- olive oil to drizzle
- sea salt & black pepper to taste

DIRECTIONS:

1. Start by threading your basil, cheese and tomatoes together on small skewers. Dash with oil before seasoning with salt and pepper. Serve immediately.

NUTRITION: Calories: 46 Carbs: 1g Fat: 3g Protein: 0g

DESSERT RECIPES

96. Almond Cookies

Preparation Time: 5 minutes

Cooking Time: 10 minutes

Servings: 4-6

INGREDIENTS:

- ½ cup sugar
- 8 tablespoons (1 stick) room temperature salted butter
- 1 large egg
- 1½ cups all-purpose flour
- 1 cup ground almonds or almond flour

DIRECTIONS:

1. Preheat the oven to 375°F. Using a mixer, cream together the sugar and butter. Add the egg and mix until combined.
2. Alternately add the flour and ground almonds, ½ cup at a time, while the mixer is on slow.
3. Once everything is combined, line a baking sheet with parchment paper. Drop a tablespoon of dough on the baking sheet, keeping the cookies at least 2 inches apart.
4. Put the single baking sheet in the oven and bake just until the cookies start to turn brown around the edges for about 5 to 7 minutes.

NUTRITION: Calories 604 Fat 36g Carbs 63g Protein 11g

97. Baklava and Honey

Preparation Time: 40 minutes

Cooking Time: 1 hour

Servings: 6-8

INGREDIENTS:

- 2 cups chopped walnuts or pecans
- 1 teaspoon cinnamon
- 1 cup of melted unsalted butter
- 1 (16-ounce) package phyllo dough, thawed
- 1 (12-ounce) jar honey

DIRECTIONS:

1. Preheat the oven to 350°F. In a bowl, combine the chopped nuts and cinnamon. Using a brush, butter the sides and bottom of a 9-by-13-inch inch baking dish.
2. Take off the phyllo dough from the package and cut it to the size of the baking dish using a sharp knife.
3. Put one sheet of phyllo dough on the bottom of the dish, brush with butter, and repeat until you have 8 layers.
4. Sprinkle ⅓ cup of the nut mixture over the phyllo layers. Top with a sheet of phyllo dough, butter that sheet, and repeat until you have 4 sheets of buttered phyllo dough.
5. Sprinkle ⅓ cup of the nut mixture for another layer of nuts. Repeat the layering of nuts and 4 sheets of buttered phyllo until

all the nut mixture is gone. The last layer should be 8 buttered sheets of phyllo.

6. Before you bake, cut the baklava into desired shapes; traditionally this is diamonds, triangles, or squares. Bake the baklava for about 1 hour just until the top layer is golden brown.

7. While the baklava is baking, heat the honey in a pan just until it is warm and easy to pour.

8. Once the baklava is done baking, directly pour the honey evenly over the baklava and let it absorb it, about 20 minutes. Serve warm or at room temperature.

NUTRITION: Calories 1235 Fat 89g Carbs 109g Protein 18g

98. Baked Apples with Walnuts and Spices

Preparation Time: 10 minutes

Cooking Time: 45 minutes

Servings: 4

INGREDIENTS:

- 4 apples
- ¼ cup chopped walnuts
- 2 tablespoons honey
- 1 teaspoon ground cinnamon
- ¼ teaspoon ground nutmeg
- ¼ teaspoon ground ginger
- Pinch sea salt

DIRECTIONS:

1. Preheat the oven to 375°F. Cut the tops off the apples and then use a metal spoon or a paring knife to remove the cores, leaving the bottoms of the apples intact.

2. Place the apples cut-side up in a 9-by-9-inch baking pan. Stir together the walnuts, honey, cinnamon, nutmeg, ginger, and sea salt.

3. Put the mixture into the centers of the apples. Bake the apples for about 45 minutes until browned, soft, and fragrant. Serve warm.

NUTRITION: Calories: 199 Carbohydrates: 41g Protein: 5g Fat: 5g

99. Red Wine Poached Pears

Preparation Time: 10 minutes

Cooking Time: 45 minutes + 3 hours to chill

Servings: 4

INGREDIENTS:

- 2 cups dry red wine
- ¼ cup honey
- Zest of ½ orange
- 2 cinnamon sticks
- 1 (1-inch) piece fresh ginger
- 4 pears, bottom inch sliced off so the pear is flat

DIRECTIONS:

1. In a pot on medium-high heat, stir together the wine, honey, orange zest, cinnamon, and ginger.

2. Bring to a boil, stirring occasionally. Lessen the heat to medium-low and then simmer for 5 minutes to let the flavors blend.

3. Add the pears to the pot. Cover and simmer for 20 minutes until the pears are tender, turning every 3 to 4 minutes to ensure even color and contact with the liquid.

4. Refrigerate the pears in the liquid for 3 hours to allow for more flavor absorption. Bring the pears and liquid to room temperature.

5. Place the pears on individual dishes and return the poaching liquid to the stove top over medium-high heat.

6. Simmer for 15 minutes until the liquid is syrupy. Serve the pears with the liquid drizzled over the top.

NUTRITION: Calories: 283 Carbohydrates: 53g Protein: 1g Fat: 1g

100. Vanilla Pudding with Strawberries

Preparation Time: 10 minutes

Cooking Time: 10 minutes + chilling time

Servings: 4

INGREDIENTS:

- 2¼ cups skim milk, divided
- 1 egg, beaten
- ½ cup sugar
- 1 teaspoon vanilla extract
- Pinch sea salt
- 3 tablespoons cornstarch

- 2 cups sliced strawberries

DIRECTIONS:

1. In a small bowl, whisk 2 cups of milk with the egg, sugar, vanilla, and sea salt. Transfer the mixture to a medium pot, place it over medium heat, and slowly bring to a boil, whisking constantly.

2. Whisk the cornstarch with the ¼ cup of milk. In a thin stream, whisk this slurry into the boiling mixture in the pot. Cook until it thickens, stirring constantly. Boil for 1 minute more, stirring constantly.

3. Spoon the pudding into 4 dishes and refrigerate to chill. Serve topped with the sliced strawberries.

NUTRITION: Calories: 209 Carbohydrates: 43g Protein: 6g Fat: 1g

101. Mixed Berry Frozen Yogurt Bar

Preparation Time: 10 minutes

Cooking Time: 0 minutes

Servings: 8

INGREDIENTS:

- 8 cups low-fat vanilla frozen yogurt (or flavor of choice)
- 1 cup sliced fresh strawberries
- 1 cup fresh blueberries
- 1 cup fresh blackberries
- 1 cup fresh raspberries
- ½ cup chopped walnuts

DIRECTIONS:

1. Apportion the yogurt among 8 dessert bowls. Serve the toppings family style, and let your guests choose their toppings and spoon them over the yogurt.

NUTRITION: Calories: 81 Carbohydrates: 9g Protein: 3g Fat: 5g

CONCLUSION

Thank you for reaching the end of this book, Mediterranean Diet Cookbook for Beginners.

I do hope that you found it enjoyable.

Before we end let me give you some more tips in maintaining and adhering to Mediterranean Diet:

1. As a reader you might have observed that the Mediterranean diet is quite similar to other types of diets like Atkins Diet, Ketogenic diet and Paleo diet. The main difference that exists between these diets is the kind of food that is used for preparation in each diet. The Mediterranean diet uses large amount of green and leafy vegetables and less of carbohydrates when compared to the other diets.

2. As you might have observed in the story, the health benefits of such a diet only remains noticeable when you completely abandon processed foods. This diet requires you to completely avoid eating any kind of processed food products.

3. As long as you follow the above-mentioned guidelines and rules of the Mediterranean diet, you will surely enjoy a healthier and a happier life.

The Mediterranean Diet is a diet that is designed to prevent you from heart diseases, heart strokes ailments, diabetes, asthma, cancer and other human ailments that are observed regularly among individuals. Using Mediterranean diet, you will be able to enjoy a better lifestyle

It is important that you realize that the Mediterranean diet is a way of life that includes a lot of food sources that you have to embrace and live with in order to enjoy the health benefits associated with it. When you follow Mediterranean diet, you are guaranteed to enjoy a better lifestyle. This book is based on this great idea and is not a diet prescription.

As you might have noticed if you have been through the book you can receive unlimited freedom in eating the way you want as long as you are following the principles and guidelines of this great diet.

So, this book makes a full guide to the Mediterranean Diet and all the details you need to keep it at bay. So, have a great time with this book.

You also need to keep in mind that Mediterranean Diet is not a new diet, it has been followed since decades.

Therefore, if you want to reap the benefits of Mediterranean diet you have to follow some basic and thoroughly known tips provided by the book.

You are very welcomed to do rereading of the book and enjoy the information it has to offer.

With regards to the recipes in this book, I hope that you had already tried most of it and from your evaluations that most of them have to be tried for at least once. I would be glad to have contribution from you, if you have new recipes that you have developed from time to time.

The information I have provided is basic and enough to keep you on track.

I do hope that you found this book very helpful and you decide to use it as a reference in starting your own diet.

Thank you and I hope you enjoy a great day.